every
WOMAN'S
GUIDE *to* PERSONAL
POWER

WENDIE PETT

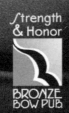

Strength
& Honor

BRONZE
BOW PUB

"You will LOVE this training system because it simply works! Wendie Pett leads you to a sexier, sculpted figure without the need for time-consuming trips to the gym. Her bright smile, motivating physique, and words of encouragement will inspire you to achieve your true God-given potential."

—Aaron Tabor, M.D.

every **WOMAN'S GUIDE** *to* **PERSONAL POWER**

The *Transformetrics™ Training System* is a trademark that is the exclusive property of Bronze Bow Publishing.

ISBN 1-932458-09-3

Published by Bronze Bow Publishing Inc.,
2600 E. 26th Street, Minneapolis, MN 55406.

You can reach us on the Internet at www.bronzebowpublishing.com

Literary development and cover/interior design by
Koechel Peterson & Associates, Inc., Minneapolis, Minnesota.

Manufactured in the United States of America

Table of Contents

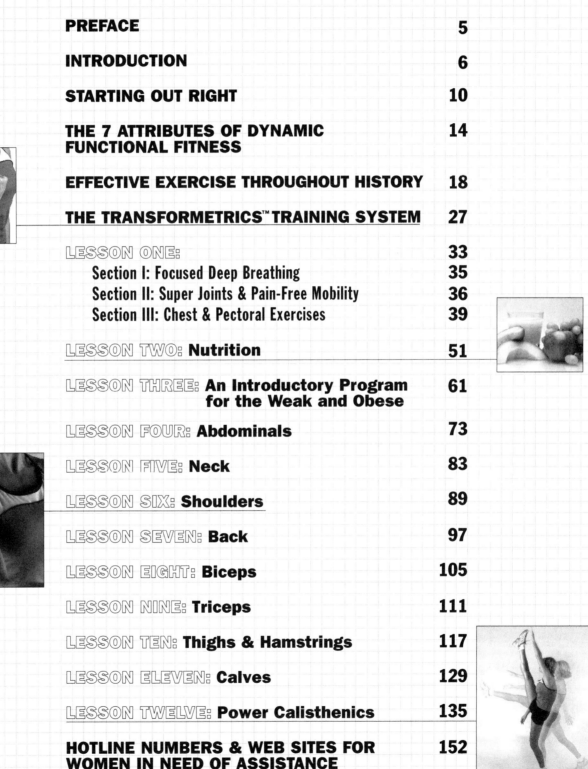

Acknowledgments

For my son, Keegan. You are my sunshine and my main motivation for wanting to live a healthier, longer life. May you learn through this book to keep your temple in good health to achieve your life's mission completely.

To the love of my life, for showing continual support and enthusiasm on this project. You continue to take my breath away. Thanks for placing all bets on me.

My family and friends, I want you to know that you have *all* played an important role with your endless encouragement and motivation while turning my vision into a reality. Thanks for always being there!

John Peterson, I couldn't have done this without you. You have been a tower of support and an incredible friend not only with this project but with life's details and struggles. You have a vision and heart like none other I have ever witnessed. Thanks for accepting everyone for who they are and only noticing the good qualities that shine through.

Tom Henry, you have an amazing talent as you capture the essence of everything you see through the camera's eye. Thanks for getting these shots done in record time while adding a little humor along the way.

Gregory Rohm, your design capabilities have sky-rocketed since I first met you. Your time and devotion hasn't gone unnoticed, and I am grateful for your talents and fun attitude on this project.

Lance Wubbels, thank you for your dedicated time on this project and all the wonderful things that your masterful literary gifts have brought to the table for Bronze Bow Publishing.

Dave Koechel and Duff Smith, for both of your positive attitudes on this project and allowing me to minister something I am passionate about to the people of God through Bronze Bow Publishing. You are both very special.

Rock, Pam, Jen, and Nells. What can I say? A girl's got'ta have gal pals to lean on. Thanks for keeping me sane!

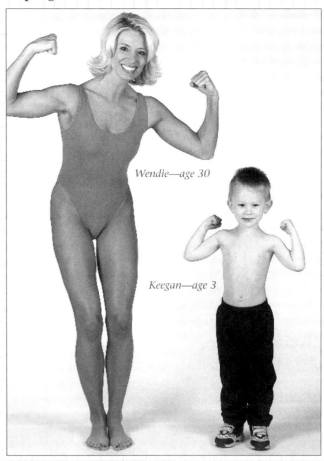

Wendie—age 30

Keegan—age 3

*I*n today's hectic world, a constant reminder of your next appointment flashes on your computer screen, beeps in your palm pilot, and dings on your watch. So many places to be and things to do, but the reality is that there are only 24 hours in a day to accomplish all that needs to be done.

But just because the world is getting busier doesn't mean that we can afford to neglect our bodies. The fact is that you may not have the time to do what you have considered your "normal workout" at the gym. However, that doesn't mean you can't transform your workout into one that allows you to exercise anytime and anyplace. You probably don't realize that you have always had the capabilities along with the built-in equipment. My goal is to show and teach you how to create an amazing sculpted body with a system that really works!

If I told you that by using your own body's resistance alone, you could build the body of your dreams, would you believe me? And that you will drastically improve your strength, flexibility, endurance, aesthetics, balance, speed, and coordination. And that you would never need to return to the gym again. And that it will cost *nothing*. And that you can start *now*. Would you believe me?

If your answer is "no," don't worry. I was a firm skeptic, too, until I broke down (literally…story to follow) and tried the *Transformetrics™ Training System* by John Peterson. It took me a week to realize I would never go back to a gym again. *Transformetrics™* worked like a dream come true. With its complete flexibility, it allowed me to continue my busy lifestyle and get a more effective daily workout than I had ever gotten before.

Still doubting? Well, I hope you're willing to take the challenge and be amazed for yourself. I have written *Every Woman's Guide to Personal Power* to be your personal instruction manual to a body transformation you're going to love!

These Exercises Are for You

Every Woman's Guide to Personal Power is for any woman, man, girl, or boy who wants to create a sleek, strong, sculpted body without having to go to the gym and lift weights to get the results they are looking for.

Transformetrics™ is the ultimate exercise system for people with busy lives, particularly for women and men who have families and seem to be always on the go. It's for the busy traveler, the fittest of the fit, and the not so fit. It's designed for anyone who wants to make a change for good health and incredible strength benefits.

Here are some of the many benefits I received from the *Transformetrics™ Training System:*

1. **A quick recovery** from a shoulder injury.

2. **A dramatic increase in strength and flexibility** in my upper and lower back. For me, that increase reduced my back pain at night to zero…and made such an improvement on my quality of sleep.

3. **It enhanced my sleep patterns** and helped me deal with stress in a more positive way.

4. **My waistline got much smaller** and more toned. (A needed gift, especially after having a child!)

Introduction

Meeting John Peterson

I thank God daily that I have had the pleasure of becoming a great friend of John Peterson, author of *Pushing Yourself to Power* and creator of the *Transformetrics™ Training System*. Without his encouragement and knowledge of how to train the *Transformetrics™* way, I would still be burning out on my old time-intensive workout and still grasping for every last bit of energy to keep going. Because of John, those days are a fading memory.

Plus, because of *Transformetrics™* I am no longer a slave to the gym and can do the exercises whenever I feel like it throughout the day. Got'ta love that!

Transformetrics™ first helped me in the rehabilitation of my injured shoulder, but John assured me that I'd also shed some unwanted flab, get fit, and feel fantastic. My life is too busy not to have the energy that I was lacking. Fortunately, my injury forced me to reflect on my lifestyle and how I exercised. These two important aspects of my life were almost constantly at war with each other, and I was ready for a transformation. John led the way!

My Family

My parents and younger sister live in Lewisville, Texas. I grew up in a normal home (well, depending on your definition of *normal*) and had the most loving parents anyone could ever ask for. My father has put in over thirty-five years at Ford Motor Company, and my mother worked for over thirty years at AAFES (Army and Air Force Exchange Service). My sister and I were both active in dance and school sports, and staying in shape was a part of our daily

lives. Obviously, my parents worked extremely hard to give us a fulfilled life, and we are so fortunate to have wonderful supportive parents.

Growing up in Texas as one of the only two girls my age on the block, I was something of a tomboy. My neighborhood was full of boys, and I was fortunate they let me become a regular player in their tackle football, dodge ball, and soccer games. One might think they wouldn't be as rough when they tackled "a girl" carrying a football, but that assumption would be wrong. I think they all viewed me, at that age, as just one of the guys. Although I came home regularly with scrapes, cuts, and bruises, I had to remain tough or I wouldn't have anyone to play with. I certainly wasn't going to stay inside and play with dolls!

"Wait Until You've Had a Child!"

If age and gravity don't get to your body first, then just wait and see what happens if and when you have children. To put it mildly, carrying and delivering a baby tends to cause seismic shifts to one's body shape. I was one of the fortunate ones. My jeans actually fit after giving birth to my son, Keegan, but they fit in a much different way. Though I weighed the same as before I got pregnant, things had shifted a bit. Since I started training with *Transformetrics™*, my jeans fit like they should again, and my body has "shifted back" to an even better physique. Again, my thanks go out to John, more than he'll ever know.

"A woman's life can really be a succession of lives, each revolving around some emotionally compelling situation or challenge, and each marked off by some intense experience." —Wallis Simpson

How I Got Started

As I've matured, that same tomboy from my youth comes out when there is any form of competition or sport. And while a competitive nature can be used in very positive ways, it can get you into trouble as well. Trouble for me came on February 11, 2003—a day still shrouded in infamy.

Two dear friends of mine, Paul and Jenny, were taking me on a fifty-five-mile snowmobile trip outside of Hinkley, Minnesota (a small town about an hour and a half north of downtown Minneapolis). It was a beautiful, sunny winter's day. (Okay, it was downright freezing at –15°F without the windchill.) At that time, Paul was a prospective client, and he had offered that we could use his three snowmobiles. Paul had tried to arrange this trip on numerous occasions, and we couldn't back down just because it was cold. After all, we live in Minnesota, where you have to suck it up and act like a trooper! Besides, my best friend, Jenny, assured me that I would stay warm inside the snowmobile gear along with the hand and feet warmers on the sled.

We took off down the trail and soon were having a great time, enjoying the scenery and actually forgetting that we were freezing our buns off. Around lunchtime we stopped, and Paul whipped out a blue canvas and set it up like a mini-tent to block the chilling wind. Then he proceeded to make a much appreciated campfire (must have been a Boy Scout). While we warmed up and Paul cooked us a little lunch, the wind and snow really started to pick up. Unfortunately for Mr. Wind and Ms. Snow, they weren't invited to our party, so we packed up quickly and headed back to our car.

Paul took the lead, I followed, and Jenny slowly hugged the trails behind us. I kept looking over my shoulder to make sure I could see her head-light flicker from time to time as reassurance that she was on her way and safe. We stopped occasionally to close the gap a bit. After our last stop, it was only about a mile more to the car. Paul gave his sled a squeeze on the gas and sped away like a rocket.

Here is where my competitive nature got the best of me. I thought, *If Paul can speed away like that then so can I—looks like fun!* Off I roared, my tomboy taking over, who had obviously forgotten that I was a native Texan and only been on a snowmobile two previous times. And the speed was super fun…until I hit a huge chunk of ice and the sled went out of control. Although I went off the trail, I thought I could regain control if I held tight. The next thing I knew, I hit a culvert and my body crashed against the throttle. Traveling at fifty-five miles per hour my sled and I went airborne. On impact I was ejected from the sled and slammed into a tree. The tree did not budge.

At least that is what I was told. I was knocked unconscious for what seemed like several minutes (it was only seconds). Waking up to Jenny's voice saying, "Wendie, can you hear me? Can you talk? Don't move," really freaked me out. I was absolutely freezing and hurting badly—my arm wouldn't move. Paul rode off to get the car while we waited. Jenny was so sweet to lie down next to me in the snow and try to keep me warm and calm.

Seeing my sled upside down, the windshield lying several yards away, and one of my snow boots several more yards away, a couple of very sweet ladies in a car stopped to help. Before I knew what was going on, the ladies ran home, called an ambulance, and brought back a pile of blankets to keep me warm. It's nice to know that compassion still exists. I wish I knew who they were so I could thank these heavenly angels.

The ambulance arrived just as Jenny helped me to my feet and at the same time that Paul arrived with the car. I decided to go with Paul and Jenny, and they took me to the Pine City Urgent Care. After being examined, I found out I had severely broken my clavicle and injured my leg near my shin. Naturally, my emotions were running wild. I was grateful to God that I hadn't hit the tree an inch or so to the left as I would have hit my head. But I was also upset because I had an important sales trip planned for the following day to Denver with John Peterson. I even thought of my dance competitions, which were less than three months away.

I called to tell John about the accident, but I said I could still go on the trip to Denver. Personally, given my injury, I think John was amused that I was determined to go. He told me to just rest and he would call to see how I was feeling in an hour or so. An hour passed and John called to say, "Wendie, I'm way ahead of you on this one. I've already made arrangements and rescheduled our appointment for two weeks from now…if you are feeling better by then."

Transformetrics™ to the Rescue

The clavicle is the long curved bone that connects the upper part of the breastbone with the shoulder blade at the top of each shoulder. I had to relearn how to dress myself, bathe, and take care of my two-and-a-half-year-old with just one arm. But in two weeks I was ready to fly to our business meeting.

While on the plane I talked to John about my orthopedic specialist's advice about my injuries. The doctor said there would be no way to dance in three months. The thought of not being able to dance really upset me as I had worked so hard to be able to perform with my class. I asked John, "Do you have any idea how important this dance competition is to me?"

"Of course, I do, Wendie," John said. "And the doctor would be right if you try to train in the typical way. The compression caused by the use of weights will never allow your tendons, ligaments, and bones to heal." And then he looked me straight in the eye and said, "But my *Transformetrics*™ *Training System* can have you in better shape than ever."

At first I said to myself, "You pompous jackass. The doctors tell me I can't even train, and instead of expressing sympathy you tell me the system you developed can have me ready for the competition! Just who do you think you are, Charles Atlas?" Then it dawned on me, he did! He really did! He believed he was the new "Charles Atlas" with a mission for God's people, and he was serious. I felt a flash of embarrassment and hoped that he didn't pick up on what I was thinking. Then without even consciously thinking about it, I heard myself asking, "How soon can we start?"

John just smiled, laughed a little, and said, "Wendie, with a question like that, we've already begun. As soon as the white of your eyes looks white instead of blood red, we'll start the physical exercises. For now, I need to teach you the philosophy and reasons why my system is superior to all others. But before I do, here's something my grandfather used to tell me that always served as a catalyst to get me moving in the right direction. He said, 'A wise man can profit under any circumstance, but fools lose even in the best of conditions.' Bottom line, Wendie, every trial can be a blessing if you learn the lesson it brings. So…let's learn the lessons."

Although I had seen his book and recognized his incredible physique, I was completely skeptical of a workout method that didn't use weights. Actually, I didn't understand the dynamics of *Transformetrics*™. But I had tried every type of fitness training from circuit training to body pump class, and I thought I knew what worked. At the time I had just started to see a difference during a body pump class. Body pump is basically a class that is based on high repetitions while using a bar with weights. You increase your weights as you feel comfortable, and you work all the muscle groups during this 60-minute class. You even do clean and presses. But it was killing my lower back and knees.

I asked John, "At what point should I start trying *Transformetrics*™? The pain is amplified if I even move my arm an inch, and I can feel and hear the bones popping and rubbing together, which really freaks me out."

John said, "Read about the exercises and become familiar with them. I bet in about another week you'll be able to move 50 percent more than you can right now as the bones, muscles, tendons, and ligaments are working overtime to heal your injury. At that point, if it feels ready, try to do a few contractions such as the Biceps Curl. Since you keep your arm to your side, this should be fairly pain free. Next, I would try Deltoid Shoulder Rolls and Raises. Remember, you won't be able to do these full out. Go slow and listen to your body. If it hurts, *stop!* Eventually, I want you to work up to the McSweeney High Reaches. These helped me heal my shoulder, and I had my injury for over twelve years. I ought to know what works and what doesn't. It works! Listen, kid, try *Transformetrics*™ and it will prove itself."

So, I followed John's advice, and it worked precisely as he said. After a month or so I was able to regain the upward motion of my arm. And slowly I was able to regain my strength and much more. Not only did I do the dance competition, but I was so sold on John's system that I wrote this book!

The *Transformetrics*™ Way

If I can train the *Transformetrics*™ way, then anyone who is willing and able can! I am a wife, mother, full-time career woman, author, dancer, and volunteer. My job requires traveling from time to time, and I entertain clients once or twice a week. I know what hectic means.

Going to the gym for even a quick 30 to 45 minute workout routinely took two hours out of my day. Consider a drive time of 10 to 15 minutes each way was 30 minutes down the drain. Then it took time to put my son into the daycare, which I have to pay for. Are you starting to get the picture?

Why go somewhere else when you can have a more effective and less stressful workout right in your own home. I even do these exercises while chatting with my son. He likes to try and do them with me, so we make it fun! My training consists of working out throughout the day. I even take advantage of "still time." For example, while I'm curling my hair in the morning, I'll do concentrated squats or leg curls. While driving in the car, butt squeezes and abdominal contractions are in order. Where there is a will there is a way.

You just need to be ready to make a change, and I know you can do it! With power comes confidence and vice versa.

"The key to living a healthy, happy life is not only the obvious of eating right and training the Transformetrics™ way, but seven hugs a day along with laughing until your stomach aches."

—Wendie Pett

Starting Out Right

Your Current Physical Condition

Before beginning *any* exercise program, you should always consult with a physician. Even if you feel great, it is of utmost importance that you make certain that your primary health care professional has given you a clear bill of health.

Body Types

Whenever I talk with someone about their body, I start with this advice: I believe that you need to accept the person you are and make the most of the body you have. Everyone has positive features, and I will show you how to enhance those. And everyone has negative features, which we'll try to eliminate or balance out. Beauty can be found in *everyone,* no matter what your body type. God accepts and loves each of us for who we are, and that's the bottom line. I think He's even more pleased if we keep ourselves healthy and in good shape so He doesn't have to worry about us as much. With 64 percent of the population either obese or overweight, we have room to work with most people who need exercise guidance.

Dr. William H. Sheldon wrote a fascinating book in 1954 called the *Atlas of Men.* He studied and defined hundreds of different body types, or somatotypes. For our purposes, I am limiting our discussion to four body types: apple, tubed, hourglass, and pear shaped. The goal is to identify the somatotype you were born with.

Tube Shape. Bust, waist, and hips are similar in width. An undefined waist—in other words, a straight up and down look. Little to no curves. The body type most envied by other women.

Apple Shape. Full bust, waist, and upper back. Carry more weight around your abdomen. Back

end is pretty flat and small. In other words, "no junk in the trunk."

Hourglass Shape. Shoulders and hips are similar in width. A well-defined waist. The body type most envied by other men.

Pear Shape. Hips are wider than shoulders and bust. A well-defined waist and a shapely back side. Think of a J.Lo body.

Examine the shapes carefully and decide which category is yours. The beauty of *Transformetrics*™ is that all the exercises in this book work to shape the entire body, no matter what your somatotype. It also allows you to work on any "trouble zones" that you may want to reshape.

I fall into the tube-shape category. During my teenage years I remember getting teased all the time. I hated my shape and was ashamed to wear skirts along with sleeveless shirts for fear that people would make fun of my "stick legs and arms." Boys used to tease me that my shoulder blades were bigger than my breasts, and they said they couldn't tell if I was coming or going. Talk about going home and crying on my mother's shoulder. I was mortified. Today, I laugh when looking back at the way I let others get to me. Shoot, I'm still not sure that my shoulder blades aren't about the same size as my chest. But I am comfortable with that now! Hopefully, you will learn to love who you are and only enhance your God-given shell.

> *"If you think you can, you're right; and if you think you can't, you're right."*—Mary Kay Ash

Exercise Duration

I would suggest you commit to a time frame of about 30 to 45 minutes a day. This doesn't mean that you have to do all 30 to 45 minutes at one given time. If I wake up late, I may only do a 10-minute workout at home and then make up for it throughout the day—whether it's on my break, between appointments, or once I get home. I make sure I fit the exercises into my schedule, and I don't let my workouts run my schedule. I'm not as stressed or disappointed in myself if I didn't do my workout first thing in the morning because I have the rest of the day to fit it in at some point and time. It's great!

Flexibility is freedom for me, and it can be yours, too. Also, by exercising throughout the day, you challenge your metabolism and burn more calories than when you work out at one specific time of the day.

The Most Important Exercises

John Peterson calls these the *Dynamic Three*. They are the Furey Push-up, the Furey Squat, and the Atlas Push-up. I am going to add the Panther Stretch to these dynamic exercises to make a *Dynamic Four*.

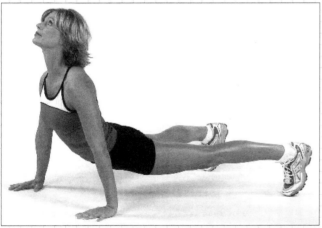

The Panther Stretch

At the Bronze Bow Publishing web site, there is an extensive forum that has generated a tremendous amount of discussion about the *Transformetrics™ Training System*. I especially enjoyed a testimonial that was written by one of the forum members, Howard Wallace. The Panther Stretch was one of the exercises that helped rehabilitate a reoccurring back injury

Howard battled. While he was utilizing five exercises, he said, "The dramatic improvement occurred during the Panther Stretch. The Panther Stretch allowed me to gradually back up farther and farther each rep. I was happy to discover the therapeutic effect of that particular exercise on my back."

I am thankful that this stretch helped Howard and could help many other people with the same need. Remember that every person is different and may respond more to certain *Transformetrics™* exercises than others. The key is to *always* listen to your body and the way it reacts to each exercise. Howard could have continued the Furey Push-ups although they were hurting him, but he was smart and listened to his body and found an alternative that fit his needs.

It took me a while to really get the feel and truly find a comfort zone while doing these exercises. So, if you don't understand the *Dynamic Three/Four* right away, don't be discouraged. Practice makes perfection. It helps to learn the exercises by using a floor-to-mid-wall-length mirror and watch yourself through the bends and stretches of each move. You will start to feel comfortable with each exercise and should continue to use the mirror as a guide. Remember to take baby steps…it's not a race.

"A journey of a thousand miles starts with a single step"—Confucius

Minimums and Maximums

On the Bronze Bow Publishing web site forum for *Pushing Yourself to Power*, minimums and maximums come up often. As a society we have been trained by all levels of athletes that in order to see results from a workout, you need to know how many sets and repetitions to do for each muscle group. In the *Transformetrics™*

Training System, you do not need to count sets or reps. Your body will tell you when to move on to the next muscle group rather than a number in a sequential count.

But since we are programmed to count reps, I have included suggested "sets and reps" of what I do (although I may vary from day to day). I let my body tell me when it's ready to be pushed or if it is still in its reconstruction phase. The way that Dynamic Visualized Resistance (DVR) and Dynamic Self-Resistance (DSR) exercises work is by mastering and maintaining your focus of mind over muscle.

Here's what I mean by mind over muscle. Picture yourself with a five-pound dumbbell in your hand, then bend your arm as though you are doing a Bicep Curl. Now picture a ten-pound dumbbell and do the same. Now a fifteen-pound dumbbell and repeat the exercise. Do you feel the tension in your bicep? If you don't, then you weren't thinking into the muscle and your training will have to start here.

The intensity of every exercise I perform actually allows me to do fewer repetitions and fewer sets of each exercise. As you become stronger and apply more force, your body cries out for fewer reps and sets, not more. You will physically be exhausted if you don't listen to the needs of your body and will be training only for your body to respond in the opposite manner.

"Transformetrics™ is about training smarter, not longer or harder."—John Peterson

With increased intensity, you might wonder about injury. The amazing thing about this system of exercise is it was constructed to protect against injury as well as heal old injuries. How, you may ask? Well, easing up on tension if you are squeezing or flexing too hard is a natural response that your body will do automatically,

and therefore there is zero room for injury. Whether you are nine or ninety, you may utilize *Transformetrics™* and see huge results.

Remember: Mind over muscle. The mind is a terrible thing to waste!

Body of Your Dreams

If you wonder if *Transformetrics™* is going to make you "Bulk like the Hulk," wonder no longer. If you perform *Transformetrics™* as I show you along with a nutritious meal plan, you will eventually have the body of a lean athlete. A *Transformetrics™* body could compare to the body and shape of dancers, gymnasts, swimmers, and even martial artists.

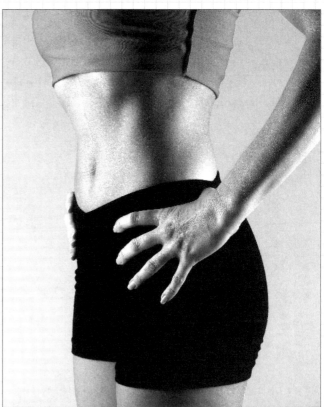

This training system can and will give you the body of your dreams as long as you follow the plan. I have created *The Power Living Journal* to help keep you motivated by journaling each exercise and nutritional goal you achieve along the way. Besides looking in the mirror and seeing the ripped muscles that have been brought to life or back to life, most us need to document our newfound strength and diet achievements. With my busy lifestyle, I find it to be very helpful. It's hard for me to keep up with every detail of my workout and diet if I don't keep a log.

Many bodybuilders have switched to this type of training method because they have found it to be just as effective but without the injuries involved with lifting heavy weights. You can build muscle mass while staying proportioned to your frame, staying lithe, super strong, and fit while doing *Transformetrics™*.

Don't wait for your body to be perfect in order for it to earn your love. It will get where you want it to be! This is a time of self-discovery that will also have many wonderful psychological benefits, so enjoy the transformation at each phase. Give this a chance to work and you'll see that this book really is *Every Woman's Guide to Personal Power*.

Helpful Tip: Trim your fingernails down so that you can make a fist comfortably to perform tension throughout each exercise. Otherwise, your nails will dig into the palm of your hand and will not allow each exercise to be performed correctly.

"With power and strength comes confidence."
—Wendie Pett

Weight Loss and Reduced Body Fat

Achieving and maintaining a healthy weight is a science as well as a personal mastery. You won't find it in a bottle or diet book or in a pill. The key is to make certain you are giving your body the right amount of nutrients to keep your weight steady and to help you feel strong and energized at the same time. Of course, regular exercise is a critical element for any successful weight-loss and weight-maintenance program. Every person is different and needs more or less of some nutrients than others. For instance, my body has a tendency to burn iron quickly, and I fatigue easily if my iron is not balanced throughout the day. I take a woman's multiple vitamin and make sure to add extra servings of "heme" iron, which is the most absorbable. You can find heme iron in leafy green vegetables, dried fruit, meat, poultry, and fish. Although I am not a vegetarian, iron deficiencies are most common in men and women who are. Don't rush to the nearest health food store in search of a supplement for any type of nutrient deficiency. Most can be maintained through diet alone.

"It is not fair to ask others what you are not willing to do yourself. You gain strength, courage, and confidence by every experience in which you really stop to look fear in the face. You must do the thing which you think you cannot do."

—Eleanor Roosevelt

The 7 Attributes of Dynamic Functional Fitness

I've read and heard the term *functional fitness* tossed around for so long that it seems to have lost whatever meaning someone originally meant by it. Here's my functional definition for *functional fitness:* being able to hold a baby in one arm and a bag of groceries in the other without feeling like I'm going to drop either one! Or being able to play rough and tumble with my son without a fear of hurting my back. It is the million and one things I do on a daily basis that require suppleness of joints and flexibility of muscle tissue and that keep my body strong and pain free.

My definition of fitness is the quality or state of being fit or suitable; well adapted; to be correctly shaped or adjusted to; in a suitable condition for doing something.

To understand what real functional fitness is to you as an individual, I will describe the way the *Transformetrics™ Training System* can help you develop functional fitness and apply it to your everyday lifestyle.

First, there are seven distinct features of dynamic functional fitness. The attributes are as follows and will be developed naturally if you follow the *Transformetrics™* way:

1. **Strength**
2. **Flexibility**
3. **Endurance**
4. **Speed**
5. **Balance**
6. **Coordination**
7. **Aesthetics**

Though I have listed the attributes in a certain order, the truth is that none is more important than another. They are equally important.

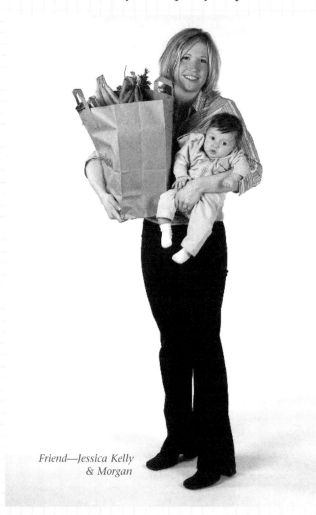

Friend—Jessica Kelly & Morgan

1. Strength

Women need strength for everything we do in life. Whether it is holding a child in an awkward position, lifting the ottoman to vacuum, shoveling snow (if you live in the frozen tundra of Minnesota), or having the strength required for self-defense purposes. You would be amazed at how strength has saved many women's lives from evil predators.

Strength does not mean that one must become muscle bound like a man. Muscles that are strong are usually pleasing to the eye. Most women want their muscles toned, firm, and defined in a feminine manner, which is precisely what *Transformetrics*™ does. You will not "bulk up" using this training system. This is not possible due to the lower level of testosterone that we have in our system compared to men. On the other hand, you can get ripped, toned, and add to your muscle mass in a natural-looking way.

2. Flexibility

Individual flexibility depends on many factors, including joint structure, ligaments, tendons, muscles, skin, fat tissue, body temperature, gender, and age. Some of my girlfriends in dance class are as flexible as rubber bands, and others have to practice stretching to get there. I believe that genetics plays a huge factor in the way your muscles were built and how pliable the tissue is.

Muscular flexibility is important in the assessment of health and overall quality of life.

I feel fortunate to have stayed fairly flexible over the years because flexibility has allowed me to play and wrestle with my son, dance, golf, and do other physical activities I love. Even life's simplest activities that you do instinctively and on a daily basis require flexibility.

Without stretching and flexibility, the connective tissue of the muscle becomes weak. That weakness increases the potential for damage when situations suddenly demand a powerful muscular contraction. A key aspect of the *Transformetrics*™ workout involves stretching both before and after the workout to prevent injury. So why after the workout? Well, after you have fatigued your muscles through the workout, your muscles retain a "pump" and are shortened somewhat. This "shortening" is mainly due to the repetition of intense muscle activity that often only takes the muscle through part of its full range motion. The "pumped" muscle is also full of lactic acid and other by-products from the exhaustive exercise. The muscle needs to be stretched afterward or it will retain this decreased range of motion as it "forgets" how to make itself as long as it can be. Stretching removes the lactic acid, reduces the tightness of the muscles, and elongates them again.

If you are working on increasing or maintaining flexibility, it's very important to take your muscles and joints through their full range of motion. (Basically, until you cry, "Uncle.") Hold the stretch for 10 seconds without bouncing through the stretch. Before you know it, you will feel like you can kick to the stars. There is a group of dancers called the Sixty Karats who have danced all over the country—average age of 78. They are flexible even at that age, and can they move! Watch out, Rockettes!

3. Endurance

Endurance is the time span between when an individual begins a physical activity and then terminates the activity because of exhaustion. It is how long you can do an activity. Whether it is chasing your kid at the park, walking to the store, waxing your car, or climbing a few flights of stairs, they all require some form of endurance.

Like anything else, you must train yourself and work your way up to increased endurance. You can improve your lung capacity and build your heart muscles to make fatigue a distant distraction by coaching your body to be pushed a little more with each endurance activity you perform. Even if it involves a simple chore or errand that you may become slightly exhausted performing, you can guide your body to respond differently over time.

Trained endurance allows long distance runners, swimmers, dancers, and many other athletes to conserve their energy over a long period of time and use it on a steady schedule, depending on the activity.

4. Speed

Speed conditioning allows an athlete to move his or her body more rapidly. Many sports and activities require speed training for maximum execution. To move faster you need to continue to build strong, well-conditioned muscles. Shortly after I started training with *Transformetrics*™, I noticed that the sprints I occasionally add on my runs got easier and much faster. It's fun to challenge yourself from time to time.

It would be nice to know that thanks to your speed conditioning you could escape a bad situation if you are ever faced with one. There are two types of speed: initial speed, which allows you to respond with a fast action, almost as a reflex; and maximum speed, which is the fastest action that your body can deliver.

Be aware of your limits and only push yourself according to your body's responses. During speed conditioning is where many athletes end up pulling and tearing muscles.

5. Balance

I have danced for most of my life, and balance is at the heart of becoming a successful dancer. You can have all the strength and speed in the world, but without balance you'll be an awkward disaster. You need balance in everything you do, not only at an athletic level. Let's face it, balance

allows us to accomplish most things easier. We have just taken for granted that balance is a built-in phenomenon and rarely put strength training in our minds as a means to help with this attribute of functional fitness. But they go hand-in-hand.

Many people actually meditate in balancing positions such as the Furey Bridge. This allows and depends on the central nervous system to work while integrating our ability to respond with the inner ear, eyes, muscles, and sensations of the lower extremities. Increased muscle strength can enhance the sense of balance and all the balance reactions.

6. Coordination

One of the most important factors that will determine whether an athlete is successful is the amount of coordination the individual possesses. The more coordinated the athlete, the better they will perform during competition.

We notice coordination early in the stages of life. A child shows coordination as a baby when they hold a rattle, roll over, crawl, walk, run, and play. Just by watching you can almost determine if your child will be a "natural" athlete or if major practice will be needed to increase the coordination of muscular skills. It's never too late to improve coordination skills—everyone can do it with the right training and frame of mind.

When you are well-coordinated, life's little tasks go smoother. Think of trying to write, brush your teeth, or even throw a ball with the opposite hand than what you usually use. This is tough for most people, while others are ambidextrous. Their coordination and motor skills are more enhanced naturally while other individuals would need to practice to accomplish such tasks. But, again, it's never too late to develop new, desired coordination.

7. Aesthetics

Aesthetics is the bottom line for why most people work out. It refers to how your body looks and how you feel about the way it looks. As a motivation tool, the power of aesthetics is amazing. We are kidding ourselves if we try to dismiss the role that perceived beauty has upon our self-image. We want to look in the mirror and feel good about the person we see.

Aesthetics in the human body is similar to aesthetics in art. We all have our own personal aesthetics by which we judge our bodies as well as art. One painting may touch our soul and be everything that we find aesthetically pleasing, while another painting that others love may not be of interest to us. We are all different and have unique ideas as to what beauty means.

However, we typically judge our bodies with immense criticism, which is partially why there is such a swelling of demand for cosmetic plastic surgery, gastric-bypass surgery, liposuction, and breast implants. We don't see what we want in the mirror, and often we jump to get it the quick way.

I know very few men or women who are truly satisfied with their bodies. *Transformetrics*™ can definitely get you there, but you need to remember that to have the body you desire you will need to make a complete, lifelong change. There is no single "quick fix" that can be done that is 100 percent safe or guaranteed. What you do with your life and your body is under your control. If you follow the tactics and strategies within the pages of this book, you will achieve your goal.

Question & Answer

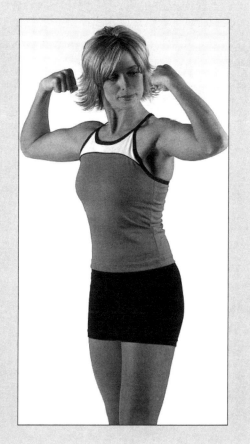

Q: I have been attending a body pump class and feel sore and wiped out all the time, though I'm seeing some positive results. If I follow your program, will it be as effective?

A: Well, from past personal experience I can relate to your question. Body pump made my lower back ache beyond belief. And my body was working on overload to repair and heal my joints, tendons, and ligaments that were affected by the added weight I applied to each exercise as instructed. *Transformetrics*™ allows you to perform the same muscle-sculpting exercises without the stress that comes from weights. You will find that *Transformetrics*™ actually is more effective because you focus and "think" into each muscle that is being developed. When I started training with *Transformetrics*™, I saw amazing results in a very short time, not to mention the delight of pain-free sleep.

Effective Exercise Throughout History

*I*t seems as though whenever I click on the television on the weekend I see a new piece of fitness equipment and a new training method. From circuit training to body pump classes, there is at least one hot new fad every year. And I've tried my share of "the latest and the best." I've invested my time and energy and hard-earned money into some programs that worked and some that didn't. But I was never satisfied. If something "better" came along, I was ready to listen and give it a try.

If you're like me, at some point you stop and ask yourself, "Why am I forever chasing and forever frustrated? When will I find a solution that works—permanently?"

Besides the fact that *Transformetrics™* worked to help heal my injured shoulder, what I found appealing about it is that people have been practicing this type of exercise method for centuries. If one looks back to the Olympians in ancient Greece, they trained their bodies to become strong sculpted masterpieces without any of the body pump classes or the newest pieces of training equipment of today. They used controlled, super slow, resistance types of movements similar to those of *Transformetrics™*.

When you study the sculptures of the physiques of the ancient Olympic athletes, you see the amazing harmony of the symmetrical bodies they produced. The *Transformetrics™ Training System* is designed to ensure the same marvelous synergy of each and every muscle group that leads to a harmonious balance between muscle size and aesthetics. The body must be trained to show that each body part has visible delineations, lines of symmetry and perfect proportions. And *Transformetrics™* delivers as no other system that I have tried or heard about.

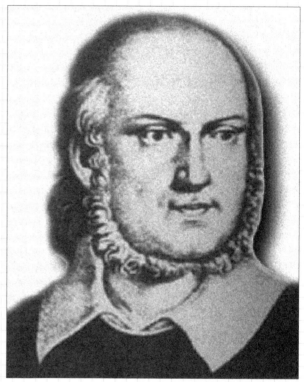

Friedrich Ludwig Jahn

In the early 1800s, Friedrich Ludwig Jahn was a pioneer of modern physical culture exercise in Germany and became the father of gymnastics. Brooding upon the humiliation of his native land by Napoleon, he conceived the idea of restoring the spirits of his countrymen by the development of their physical and moral powers through the practice of gymnastics. He helped make training easier by inventing the parallel bars, rings, balance beam, the horse, and the horizontal bar—all of which require the development of flexibility, strength, neuromuscular coordination, and cardiovascular endurance.

Jahn is noted for saying, "As long as man has got a body here below...which enervates into a vain shadow without power and strength, without endurance and persistence, without agility and skills—the art of gymnastics will have to take up a large part of human education." Unfortunately for Jahn, he fell out of favor with the government of the day. Nevertheless, his intent was to achieve the same goal of the ancient Olympians—for his people to be strong, healthy, fit, and full of energy. He proved the effectiveness of simple, controlled movements in the building of powerful physiques.

After studying the women in history who were instrumental in physical culture, I did not find many who fit the *Transformetrics*™ mold. I think this is mainly due to the lack of understanding of how a person can think into the muscle. Joyce L. Vedral, Ph.D., author of *The 12-Minute Total-Body Workout*, seemed to understand this concept. Although she used light weights, she clearly understood what you could achieve without using the heavy weights that eventually cause injury while trying to create the body of your dreams. She believes in the principles of dynamic tension and the pyramid technique to continually challenge your muscles. I believe in the same technique, minus the weights.

John Peterson, of course, is my true mentor with *Transformetrics*™. John is a veritable walking encyclopedia on the history of physical culture. John's personal story in *Pushing Yourself to Power* is worth the price of the book alone. The fact that he looks like he does today in his early 50s is amazing enough. But the fact that he contracted polio in 1956, which left his legs dreadfully misshapen, and was the target of a bully's torture is the stuff of legends. He was fortunate to have gone on to be schooled in the

Earle E. Liederman course and the Charles Atlas course, which took him from being a 94-pound weakling to the man you see today.

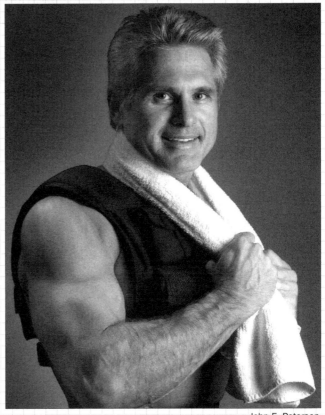

John E. Peterson

Earle Liederman was the undisputed King of the Mail-Order Bodybuilders of the late 1910s and all of the 1920s. He is probably the most instrumental person in creating America's awareness of strength and physical conditioning. Many people still feel that his original books were the most thorough and well-conceived books ever published on this subject.

The Liederman course of exercise was primarily *free hand* resistance exercises. He put a strong emphasis on the push-up as the key to upper body strength and development, and the single knee bend as the key to the lower body development. He also challenged his students to do a wide variety of chinning exercises, and he had a few exercises that required his elastic chest expander.

Utilizing a brilliant series of ads, Liederman built a huge following through offering his course via mail-order. The entire course was written so that anyone could train at home and attain the same physical development he did.

In 1917, Liederman met the young man, Angelo Siciliano, who had changed his name to Charles Atlas, and the two-men put together a vaudeville act that showcased their strength, hand-balancing skills, and physical development. Young Atlas had transformed his physique using much the same weight-resistance exercises that Liederman taught.

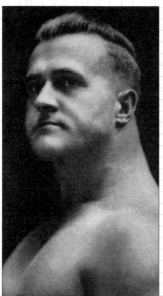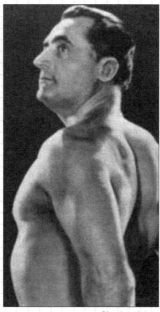

Earle E. Liederman   Charles Atlas

Atlas had learned the secret of stretching his muscles with great tension through watching the big jungle cats at the Brooklyn Zoo. Then he added hundreds of push-ups, sit-ups, and deep knee bends to develop his own physical training system.

Charles Atlas went on to become a legend, and his mail-order bodybuilding course transformed hundreds of thousands of young men from the 1930s to the 1960s. And among those thousands of students was young John Peterson, who determined at the age of ten to never allow another Goliath-like bully to beat him up. Funny that Atlas began in a similar fashion with his getting sand kicked in his face by a thug on a beach at the age of sixteen.

You will notice that I refer to the names, Liederman and Atlas, when describing certain exercises that are named after them. Unlike weightlifters who pack on massive muscle bulk, these two men were sculpted like Greek gods and could perform amazing acts of strength that men twice their size could not achieve. And yet the men trained without using weights. That may sound absurd to you, but it is the truth. The *Transformetrics™ Training System* was born out of this same philosophy that has been proven effective by many physical culturists throughout history. We live in an era dominated by weightlifting for strength, but *Transformetrics™* can deliver all the strength development you'll ever want without the stress on your joints, ligaments, tendons, and nerves that leads to injury over an extended period of time. You'll be amazed at what you can accomplish and end up being healthier than you ever thought possible.

"When training yourself, try to make exercises resulting to a healthier than physically stronger body."

—Isocrates (436–338 B.C.)

How to Get a Handle on Your Life!
FEMALE FACTS AND ISSUES

Eating Disorders—Getting Trapped in the Peer Pressure

If you've looked at any magazines or checked out *Entertainment Tonight* lately, you might have noticed that many of the movie stars look like they weigh a buck 'o nine. Reality is that most of the photos have been airbrushed and most of the movie stars have personal trainers and chefs. In a perfect world we would all be airbrushed and have personal trainers and chefs, but in the meantime we must take care of ourselves and educate ourselves on how to exercise correctly and how to eat to live. And we must refuse to get trapped in the peer pressure that leads to eating disorders.

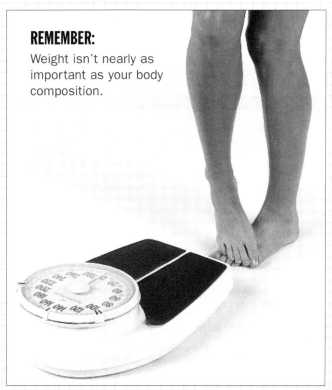

REMEMBER:
Weight isn't nearly as important as your body composition.

"Sometimes you need to step into your own shadow in order to find the light."

—Wendie Pett

Some women live to eat by bingeing. Guilt eventually sets in, which leads to purging, undereating, or the use of laxatives. This is known as *bulimia nervosa.* Bulimia *will not* help you lose weight; in fact, over time it actually has the opposite effect. To abuse the body this way leads to an out-of-control metabolism that never seems to regulate. Because a bulimic is starving her body, once she puts food into her body, no matter what it is, her body holds on to it and stores it as fat. Bulimia causes depression, mood swings, major dental problems, esophagus irritation due to the acid in the stomach from persistent vomiting, irregular heartbeat, kidney disease, and the list goes on.

Anorexia nervosa is marked by an extreme fear of becoming overweight and leads to excessive dieting to the point of serious health problems and sometimes death. Basically, an anorexic just won't eat or is very restrictive and refuses to maintain a minimally normal body weight for their height and age. Most anorexics tend to exercise constantly in fear of any type of weight gain. Most want everything in their lives to be perfect, and to them being thin is perfection. Anorexia causes girls to stop having menstrual periods, to get sick often, to have mood swings, dry skin, thinning hair, brittle bones, and far worse.

Added to bulimia and anorexia are the other types of eating disorders, such as compulsive eating, binge eating (similar to bulimia but without the purging), the over-exerciser, the diet-pill abuser, and the fad-diet abuser. All of these disorders involve one major factor—a lack of self-esteem. A person trapped in one of these disorders must first learn to love herself for who she is and not for the way she looks.

My friend Peter Lamas has applied makeup and styled hair for over three decades to supermodels and famous women such as Cindy Crawford and Princess Diana. He has found that no matter how thin, how beautiful, or how talented the woman, it never shows if her self-esteem is lacking. Health and beauty must first shine from the inside out. I almost feel that lacking self-esteem is a disorder within itself.

I have a friend (we will call Joe) who has been recovering from the pain that these diseases leave behind. Joe met a beautiful and vivacious gal (we will call her Terri) at church, and they grew strong in love. Terri had struggled with bulimia and anorexia throughout her 20s and 30s. She tried on numerous occasions to stop, but nothing worked until she went to a faith-based group where she found her acceptance through God's love. Recovered and feeling wonderful, Terri's new life really started to unfold when she met Joe. After a lengthy courtship, they sensed that God had brought them together and were united through marriage. Everything seemed to fall into place, and they were in total bliss for six months. Then Terri suffered a major coronary and was rushed to the hospital with Joe by her side. Joe felt helpless in the waiting room and prayed as he had never prayed in his life. Eventually, a doctor in a white coat delivered the news that his bride had passed away, and there was nothing they could do to save her. There might have been a chance to save her if she had not damaged all her internal organs through the past eating disorders. Joe was in total shock. Terri had never told him of her problem.

My message is that by surrendering to eating disorders you may not only die young but hurt the people you love. If you need anonymous assistance, I encourage you to go the resources listed in the back of this book that can give you guidance and professional support. I know these disorders are more common than what most people admit to, but I pray that you realize how important you are to this world and that you are loved. I hope this book will give you the edge needed to start a life worth living.

"You can rescue a woman from a dragon—because you can go slay the dragon—but you can't rescue a woman from herself."
—Laura Schlessinger

I was recently at a friend's family gathering and noticed that her younger sister and her friends were all super thin. I overheard them talking about recent fad diets and saying to one another, "I am so fat. Look at this roll." I couldn't believe it. There wasn't an ounce of fat on any of them—*zero*. They were all wearing the cute hip hugger jeans and had flat tummies, no hips, and for sure no butts. What happened to the J.Lo craze? Just kidding. Guess that's the other extreme! Anyway, these girls actually looked unhealthy in a way that their chests were semi-concaved.

I talked with the girls about eating balanced meals instead of "dieting" and explained how to gain muscle mass and strength through exercise. I showed them that *Transformetrics*™ provides the strength and energy their bodies were missing while it contributes to bone health. For women, it is very important to maintain healthy bones and avoid osteoporosis. Bone flexibility is key and can only be created and maintained through nourishment and toning the muscles around them.

Transformetrics™ enables this to happen in a non-strenuous way.

I also told the girls that I had asked 50 men and women (ages 30 to 55) what body type they preferred, and 48 out of the 50 responded that they would much rather see a woman who is physically fit with natural curves. They didn't think that being thin was bad if that was her genetic makeup and she looked healthy.

> *"Enjoying what God gave you is wonderful,*
> *but there is nothing wrong with enhancing it*
> *with strength, flexibility, and self-esteem."*
> —Wendie Pett

Osteoporosis

"Osteo" means "bone" and "porosis" means "porous." Throughout your life, your body is continually going through a bone-building cycle in which new bone replaces the broken down old bone. When 20 percent of your bone mass has been imbalanced during this cycle and not enough new bone replaces the old, you have osteoporosis. It is especially common among women that after menopause their bones become porous, break easily, and heal slowly. My grandmother suffered from this silent disease and broke her hips several times as a result. So why not control it now so you don't have to worry about becoming the next Hunchback of Notre Dame?

Here are the facts. From the age of 35 to menopause, our bone mass slowly declines. There is a gradual decrease in the production of new bone matter. Estrogen (a female hormone) helps to maintain bone strength, but estrogen declines at menopause and bones therefore become more brittle and weak. Bone mass typically peaks between the ages of 25 and 35, so treat your body right now. You may actually get tested for bone loss with a BMD—bone mineral density test—to find out if you are already at risk. Recommendations for this test are for women age 60 or over, women who have been on hormone replacement therapy for a long period of time, postmenopausal women with fractures, and all postmenopausal women under age 65 with other risk factors besides menopause.

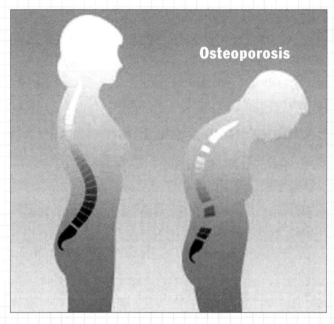

Transformetrics™ and key nutrients can significantly help you reduce your risk for osteoporosis. On top of eating the required 1,000 to 1,500 milligrams of calcium a day (depending on your age), one should boost your intake of folic acid, zinc, and iron. Half of all women in the U.S. over the age of 50 have thinning bones. Fortunately, you can take care of your bones early with *Transformetrics*™ and diet. Your bones build and maintain bone mass while performing exercises in which your bones and muscles work against gravity, such as jogging, walking, or stair climbing. The resistance training in *Transformetrics*™ helps maintain bones by strengthening the muscles around them.

Smoking and drinking too much alcohol or caffeine can also contribute to bone loss. If you are experiencing bone loss, these are habits you can curb or eliminate.

More Eskimo women have osteoporosis than any other descent and yet they get more calcium than any other nationality. Why? Lack of sunlight. We also need Vitamin D, which allows our body to absorb the calcium, and the sun is an essential source of producing Vitamin D. I am not saying to soak it up and become rawhide like the character in the movie *Something About Mary*, but a certain level of sunlight is essential. The perfect book on this is from Peter Lamas, *Sun Exposure: Its Benefits and Dangers*.

Perimenopause and Menopause

It is ironic that the menstrual period that starts in young adults leaves our lives the same way it came into it...by surprise for the most part! Well, ladies, menopause is just another fact of life and a natural part of aging. The sick joke is that we all get this at different stages and ages of our lives, and we can only approximately predict when it's going to move into our life and try taking over our internal body temperature, sleep pattern, moods (as if we are Cybil), and change our sexual desires from *yes* to *no way, get away!*

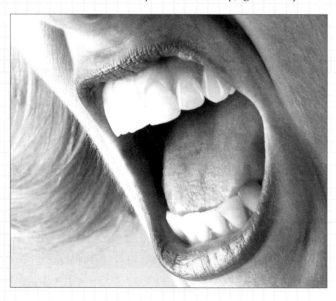

Most women, typically speaking, go through some form of ceasing of menstruation between the ages of 40 to 60. Hormone replacement therapy (ERT) is recommended by most doctors during menopausal stages, but I would recommend some natural alternatives and to use ERT as a last resort. Revival Soy is a product that has been proven to help many women subside the menopausal symptoms. I am a huge fan of natural, God-given remedies! Soy offers the richest of isoflavones that act as weak estrogen and gives relief from the symptoms caused by menopause. Epidemiological studies in Asian populations, which consume more soy than any other group, revealed low rates of menopausal symptoms, low rates of breast cancer, and low rates of osteoporosis.

Breast Cancer

I have several friends who have survived this horrible disease, and they all say the same thing: "Thank goodness I kept up with my regular clinical breast exams and mammograms so the lumps could be detected early." Having breast cancer has changed their goals in life and had a profound impact on their relationship with God.

My friend Penny is in my dance class and is a cancer survivor. She is always so positive and full of life in spite of what she has gone through. She wrote me about the shock she felt when she found the "giant" lump. The surgery and recovery. The meetings with the doctors when all the "could happens" were laid out. The chemotherapy and bald head and picking out a wig with her daughter and grandson, Carter. The prayers of her friends so full of spiritual caring. The anti-nausea medicine. Six weeks of radiation every Monday through Friday. Of how God used the return of a monarch butterfly to repeatedly speak comfort and peace so distinctly to her heart that she concluded, "Now tell me there isn't a God."

Penny also said, "I decided that exercise and eating well has to be a priority in my life." And she's lived up to that. I wish you could see her in dance class. That monarch is still very much alive and well. We obviously do not know the cards that are dealt for us, but I believe in the power of prayer, the power of love and friendship, and the power of simple gifts God sends from heaven.

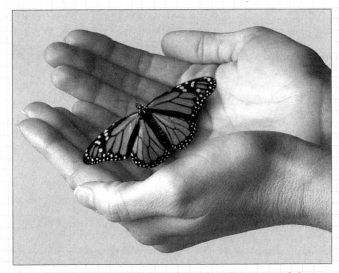

Remember to have regular checkups and learn your family health history. Women in their 20s and 30s should have a clinical breast examination as part of a periodic exam routine every three years. Note that this does not include the annual exam given by your OBGYN as well. Women age 40 and over should get a clinical breast examination by a health professional yearly along with a yearly mammogram and should continue to do so as long as they are in good health. Mammograms can miss some cancers due to its limitations, but it remains a very effective and valuable tool for decreasing suffering and death from breast cancer.

Some women who have had breast cancer and are taking medications such as Tamoxifen, Raloxifene, Toremifene, and Fulvestrant have witnessed weight gain. It hasn't been proven that these medications are the culprit for weight gain, but the women I've talked with think so. I have been asked if there are any natural remedies that do not accompany the same side effects as these medications listed above. The typical time frame to take these type of meds are five years after chemo and radiation treatments.

According to several published doctors, there seems to be growing evidence to support the use of many natural products that block the estrogen receptors just as well if not better than Tamoxifen and offer fewer side effects. One should keep animal products in their diet to a minimum, such as red meat, chicken, and dairy products, as the petrochemical compounds with estrogenic properties are concentrated in the food given to these animals, and therefore is found in the milk and fat of the meat. The deposit of these estrogens interfere in the proper utilization of production of progesterone and estrogen.

"Showing up for life. Being blessed with the rebirth that recovery brings. One day at a time."—Betty Ford

What is the ideal diet for breast cancer prevention?

High fiber, low fat (15 percent of calories).

Organic, fresh, unrefined vegetables, grains, beans, nuts, seeds, lentils, fruits, garlic, onions, kelp, flax oil, extra virgin olive oil unheated, apples, ginger, soy products, green tea, spelt, broccoli, brussel sprouts, cabbage, cauliflower, apricots, cantaloupe, carrots, millet, pink grapefruit, and yogurt.

Avoid allergenic foods, such as milk, eggs, wheat, corn, pork, beef, citrus, peanuts, and chocolate (sorry, ladies).

Try to eat 50 to 75 percent of your foods raw as the vitamins and minerals are best at this stage.

Drink 8 to 10 glasses of pure water daily.

Eliminate salts, food additives, smoked and pickled foods.

Use supplements rich in antioxidants.

Don't smoke and avoid alcohol, coffee, and tea.

Soy products are a huge success in blocking the binding of harmful xenoestrogens at the estrogen receptors. I recommend the product called Revival.

Omega-3 fatty acids have strong anti-cancer effects, and flax seed has phtyoestrogens called lignans that have been linked to breast cancer prevention.

Iodine along with selenium, zinc, and copper are important minerals for optimal thyroid function. There seems to be a link between hypothyroidism and breast cancer.

Topical progesterone cream can be used to inhibit breast cancer cell proliferation.

Heart Disease

Believe it or not, heart disease—not breast cancer—is the number-one killer among women. Cardiovascular disease claims more women's lives than the next seven causes of death combined. Over 8 million American women are currently living with heart disease. Thirty-two percent of the women who have heart disease die. African American women have a 72 percent higher risk than white women to have a heart attack or suffer from coronary artery disease. Women who smoke are at risk of having a heart attack 19 years earlier than a non-smoking woman. (Put those smoke sticks away!) *Close to*

60 percent of women have heart attacks due to a lack of physical activity or exercise. About 30 percent of the women are obese. Thirty-five percent of women who are heart attack survivors will have another attack within six years.

Grim statistics. And I think you get the point. Women need to manage their lifestyle by taking charge of their diets, exercise activity, and social crutches.

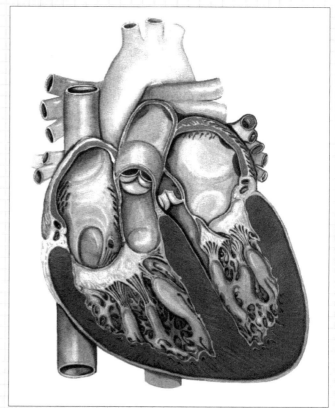

There are many heart healthy cookbooks available, but beware of fad diets. If they look too good to be true, they probably are. Just eat sensible. I define it as the 80/20 rule in chapter two on nutrition. Also be aware of your family history. Monitoring your blood glucose, blood pressure, and cholesterol helps to keep levels healthy. *Transformetrics*™ will benefit you from the outside as well as internally by helping to maintain all of these elements along with your diet.

"God always answers our prayer. Either He changes the circumstances, or He supplies sufficient power to overcome them."

—Anonymous

In this chapter I explain and outline the complete *Transformetrics™ Training System* that was developed by John Peterson in his book, *Pushing Yourself to Power*. I follow closely to John's twelve consecutive lessons, but in some of the lessons I offer more and different exercises. I focus on how to build every muscle in your body by showing you what exercises have worked in my training. And I feature more leg movements designed especially for women.

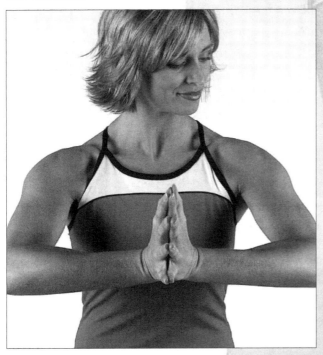

Men and women are typically in need of focusing on certain body parts that tend to be trouble zones. People have said for years that you can't "spot train," but my experience tells me that is not true. With *Transformetrics™* you can develop true overall dynamic functional fitness and at the same time focus in on your specific training needs. For instance, I created toned, lithe muscles in my arms and shoulders by actually "spot training" through *Transformetrics™*.

How John Peterson Created *Transformetrics™*

It has been fun to watch John Peterson convert his life experiences, struggles, and inspirational stories into the amazing self-help book for people of all ages and sexes, *Pushing Yourself to Power*. I have witnessed firsthand the blessings that *Transformetrics™* can deliver. The knowledge and outcome of this training system have changed my life forever. And the results I have achieved are almost impossible to put into words. I know you will feel the same.

The Criteria for the Creation of *Transformetrics™*

To put this in its simplest term—RESULTS are what *Transformetrics™* is all about! Within only a few short weeks you will be able to see astonishing development in the muscles from your neck to your toes. Every inch of your body will become sculpted in no time by incorporating high-tension exercises and maximizing each training session to its fullest.

The first step is to understand that *Transformetrics™* allows you to train your body to its highest capabilities without straining or destroying your joints, tendons, and ligaments, and without compressing your spine, draining your energy, or prematurely aging yourself. If you are looking for the fountain of youth, *Transformetrics*™ is as close as you're going to get!

One of the beautiful elements of this training system is that no equipment is required with the exception of one's own body and maybe a chair for balance or to perform dips. A bar to do pull-ups is welcomed, but a tree branch will do the trick if need be. Notice that I do not show many exercises that need these items for assistance. You can create the body of your dreams without ever using anything besides your body as your equipment.

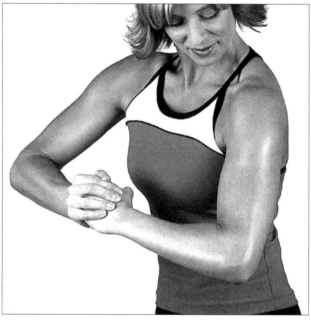

The other beautiful element about not needing equipment is that this allows you to be able to exercise virtually anytime and anywhere, making it ideal for people on the go. It allows you to work out in the privacy of your own home and can add hours to your week by not having to travel to the gym, both of which I love.

Remember, fundamentals are the basis for mastery. All advanced athletes have mastered the basics and continue to review

them with repetition. Repetition is the source of excellence, skill, and retention.

Time involved: you can get the job done with as little as 30 to 45 minutes daily. And it does not have to be consecutive minutes. Actually, I recommend that you break this time up throughout the day into 10 to 15 minute increments as this allows for maximum attention and energy on each exercise.

Variation: I show many varieties to choose from so there is zero room for boredom. It is a fact that many people terminate their workouts due to boredom alone. You won't suffer from any of that here. For example, I offer over 25 leg exercises that you can alternate on any given day and at any given time. Flexibility of choice is a wonderful thing!

Effectiveness: I have already described the healing power that *Transformetrics*™ has brought to my life. The definition in my muscles speaks for the strength factor. Am I the most ripped woman in history? No! But I reached a shape and look that I like and feel comfortable with in only a few short months, and the definition I have now is more pronounced than when I lifted weights years ago. I am in maintanance mode and will continue to perform *Transformetrics*™ as long as God allows me to live.

If you are after a look that offers bulk and mass but still sculpted and lean, you can achieve this as well. Just look at John Peterson in *Pushing Yourself to Power*. John has *never* lifted weights to build his physique, yet the power is there. You hold the key to develop your body as you wish.

Transformetrics™ is divided into four distinct categories of exercises: Isometric

Contractions, Isotonics, Joint Mobility and Flexibility, and Aerobics.

1. Isometric Contractions

What is an isometric exercise? It is an exercise that strengthens a particular muscle by tightening it, holding it, and then relaxing—all without moving the joint. Previously, I mentioned "spot training," and this is how I do it. Ultra-high tension in fixed positions against an immovable object or resistance object such as a doorway can be very effective. By contracting the muscles at their maximum force for a count of 10 or more seconds, you can dramatically increase your strength where you want it. But isometrics alone will not create the overall muscular definition you are after. You need to incorporate the other training system moves that allow full range movements for the sculpted results you desire.

Isometrics have been known to help arthritic people stay in shape without the discomfort of bending painful joints. When performed properly, isometrics have proven to increase and maintain muscle tissue to support the muscles without aggravating any of the sore, tender joints.

Isometrics not only strengthen your development, but they help develop the "mind over muscle" type of focus needed to achieve these exercises to their fullest.

2. Isotonic Exercises

Isotonic exercise is any exercise where actual movement is required. There are three categories that break up these isotonic exercises: Power Calisthenics (PC), Dynamic Self-Resistance (DSR), and Dynamic Visualized Resistance (DVR). I will walk you through each category for a clear understanding of what *Transformetrics*™ brings to the table.

Group 1: Power Calisthenics (PC).

These are specific body-weight exercises that develop your muscles in a way that every angle and direction is being maximized during each step of the exercise. They are strenuous but amazingly productive movements. I encourage you to eat your Wheaties before

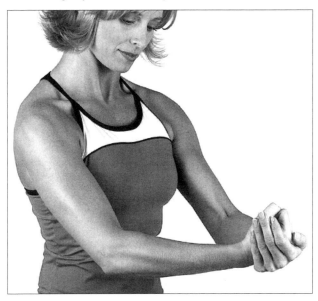

trying them on for size. You'll note that throughout the exercise sections I have labeled every exercise by its category. The (PC) designation is used on several exercises, such as the Handstand Push-up, Furey Squat, or the Furey Push-up.

Group 2: Dynamic Self-Resistance (DSR).

This grouping of exercises is defined by the fact that one muscle group resists for another. Charles Atlas and Earle Liederman were big promoters of this type of training. These exercises can be as tense as you want to make them. They prove to be very strenuous if you concentrate deeply as one limb resists the other from the start to finish of a full range of motion. I can only perform 3 to 4 repetitions of some of the DSR exercises in this book before I have exhausted the muscle group. It's amazing how little you have to do to see the results you want.

Group 3: Dynamic Visualized Resistance (DVR).

Okay, this group can sometimes seem difficult to achieve, but let me clue you in: it's easier than most people think. As you first begin to practice these exercises, you will need a mirror to watch whether you are truly visualizing, or thinking, into your muscle with every positive and negative contraction. All you need to do is literally visualize that you are working against an imaginery weight of your choice.

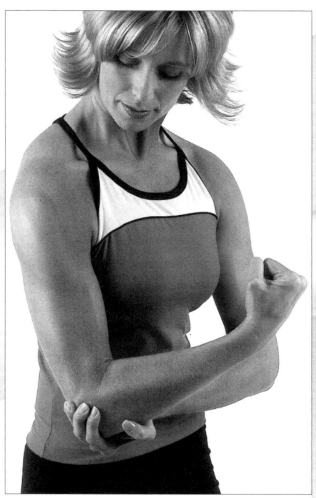

What helped me to understand the dynamics of the DVR exercises was to start with a Bicep Curl. Follow me through these steps, and you'll catch on.

First, while your right arm is down by your side, make a fist to tense the muscles from the beginning. Now imagine that in your hand is a weight (let's say it's 10 pounds). Keep a tight fist and bend your arm at the elbow, contracting with maximum force through the entire range of motion. This includes the motion on the negative or resistance part of the exercise (the motion back down to your side). If you do this movement correctly, you will have the muscles contracted at such intensity that you may see your muscles shake or vibrate. That is a good sign. It means you are doing this right and understanding how to use visualized resistance.

One of our forum members named Duff wrote us after he first started the *Transformetrics*™ program. He seemed to really get the simplicity and effectiveness of the DVR exercises right away. He said: "I love the simplicity of this system. When I was working out I always wondered why bodybuilders, who train their abs by doing crunches and gain strength and mass this way, don't train their biceps doing 'bicep crunches'? Which, of course, is what DVR is all about!"

The key is to stay focused on the entire movement without letting go of any of the tension. You may use the DVR method in just about everything you do from bending over to pick up a piece of paper to a controlled stretch exercise.

3. Joint Mobility and Flexibility

Always use the warm-up exercises in Lesson One before performing any of the *Transformetrics*™ exercises. These exercises will allow you to maintain youthful flexibility and agility without the worry of injury. If I ever feel stiff or sore from being cramped on an airline flight or sleeping in an odd position, I use the warm-up exercises to release tension and pressure. One of my favorites, which is not been pictured in this book, is to squat down with my head and arms hanging between my knees at various times throughout the day. This actually releases and stretches out the spine and leaves me feeling less sore. It looks a little funny, but it works!

4. Aerobic Exercises

Aerobics are any exercises that can be controlled for 20 minutes or longer at an intensity level that allows for a cardiovascular training effect. Most people tend to overdo their aerobic exercise, feeling that they need to get a certain "sweat on" for the exercise to have a serious impact on their fitness training. Some of them will push it so long that they end up losing muscle along the way because the body needs something to burn in place of the fat already utilized.

Most people do not need more than 20 to 30 minutes of cardiovascular training daily or even every other day for it to be effective for weight lose and all the other heart healthy benefits. People who swim, run, cycle, and even power walk have made excellent choices of aerobic activity. I have found that Furey Squats, which are found in the power calisthenics section of this book, are a great aerobic activity. If you want to feel your heart race and thighs burn, try to perform as many squats as you can within a 20-minute time frame. It's an amazing workout to say the least and will develop your legs wonderfully.

I believe the Furey Squat, Furey Push-up, Atlas Push-up, and Panther Stretch can be a mainstay in your musculature and aerobic training. They have some of the best cardio, strength, and flexibility benefits of any exercise.

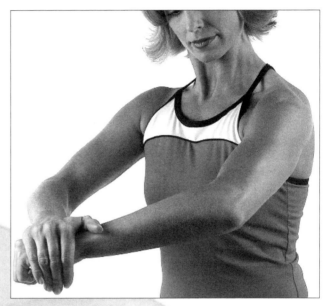

So, that's *Transformetrics*™ in a nutshell. All of which I had the fortune of learning and mastering with John Peterson. You can integrate it into the best bodybuilding system for your personal development and become the envy of your peers. Share with them your secrets so they too can enter into the functional realm of physical culture with strength and wisdom.

On to Lesson One.

Question & Answer

Q: I just found out that I'm pregnant, and I'm curious if *Transformetrics*™ is a safe way to train throughout gestation?

A: *Yes, Transformetrics*™ is safe to practice throughout your entire pregnancy. Eventually you shouldn't attempt push-ups or anything of that nature due to the growth of your belly and your equilibrium may be askew. You may use safe alternative variations, such as push-ups against the wall, to keep your program going smoothly. Studies show that when you train throughout your pregnancy it gives you the extra energy you need through all your strenuous trimesters and allows for an easier delivery.

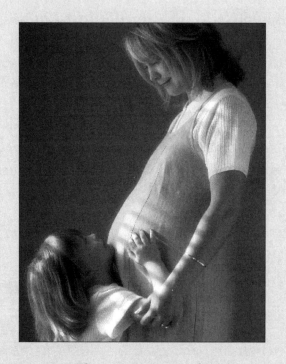

Most workout programs state that you should not attempt their program if you are pregnant and haven't been active prior to the pregnancy. The beauty of *Transformetrics*™ is that you can start out with the DVR training and begin at a comfortable tension level that does not put stress on the fetus or your body. Let's face it, pregnancy requires a woman to prepare her muscles, increase her stamina, and boost her immune system—all for the anticipation of a "natural" birth. Pregnant women who exercise reduce their possibilities of requiring a C-section, gain less weight and body fat, spend less time in labor, reduce hemorrhoids and low back pain, develop little or no varicose veins, and fatigue less frequently.

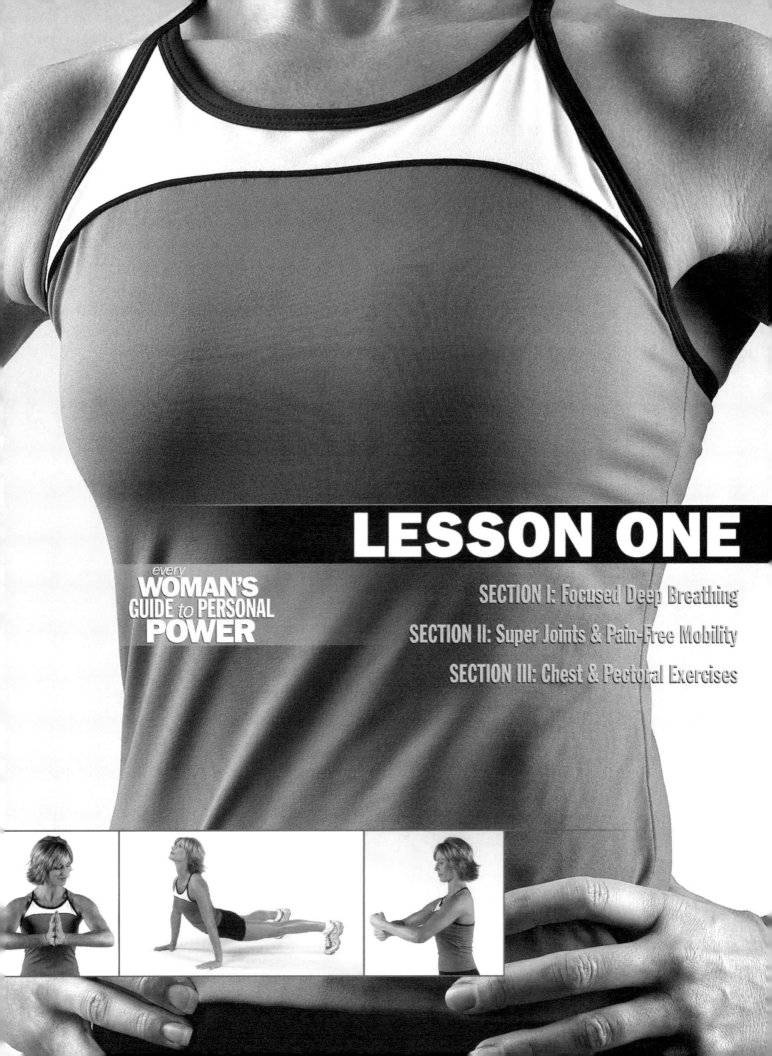

LESSON ONE

every WOMAN'S GUIDE to PERSONAL POWER

SECTION I: Focused Deep Breathing

SECTION II: Super Joints & Pain-Free Mobility

SECTION III: Chest & Pectoral Exercises

Lesson One

L esson One is the first step in the *Transformetrics™ Training System* and the most important lesson in this book. It can be incorporated by the person who is just starting a workout program for the first time in their life, and an advanced athlete can benefit from this lesson as well. I typically do this first lesson as a daily ritual at some point during the day.

If you are obese or very weak, I recommend that you first concentrate on Lessons Two and Three to learn more about nutrition, energy, and a specially designed workout that will develop your muscles and teach you how to exercise without causing stress on your joints or muscles for accidental injury to occur.

Make sure you warm up before and after your *Transformetrics™* program. It's important to loosen up the muscles and gently go through their natural full range of motion slowly. This will prepare your body for the exercises that will contract the muscles from your neck to your toes.

Every day I perform the exercises in Section I, II, and III. I alternate the remainder lessons throughout the week as I listen to my body and determine what needs to be focused on that particular day.

TRANSFORMETRICS™ SECTION I

FOCUSED DEEP BREATHING

I find that breathing is very important when doing any exercise, whether it is dancing, running, Pilates, yoga, and especially *Transformetrics™*. The primary difference with the breathing technique used while practicing *Transformetrics™* from the other exercises I listed is that it's natural breathing. You actually don't need to think or worry about when to inhale or exhale as you will naturally breathe deep while doing these exercises.

"Oxygen is your greatest and first source of energy," says Dr. Valerie Saxion in her best-selling book, *How to Feel Great All the Time*. "It is the fuel required for the proper operation of all your body systems. Only 10 percent of your energy comes from food and water; *90 percent of your energy comes from oxygen*. Oxygen gives your body the ability to rebuild itself. Oxygen detoxifies the blood and strengthens the immune system. Oxygen greatly enhances the body's absorption of vitamins, minerals, amino acids, proteins, and other important nutrients. Oxygen strengthens the heart. Increased oxygen lowers the resting heart rate and strengthens the contractions of the cardiac muscle. Correspondingly, virtually all heart attacks can be attributed to failure to deliver oxygen to the heart muscle."

Greer Childers, author of *Be a Loser*, taught how effective deep breathing can be toward weight lose and overall great health. *Prevention Magazine* has stated that deep breathing is the best solution for headaches, depression, cellulite, dropped bladder, and many other problems. The problem is that most people are starving the body of vital oxygen through their shallow breathing, according to Paul Bragg in his book *Super Power Breathing for Super Energy*. It is reported that people in Western cultures barely use one-fifth of the lung's capacity to increase the oxygen flow to their bodies.

It may be hard to believe, but deep breathing can change your life. And deep breathing is the natural way to breathe—even babies do it. When you see their tiny little chests rise up and then completely suck back in due to the use of their diaphragm, that's a deep breath. And that is how we all should breathe. It's important to take in as much oxygen as possible with every breath as well as release as much carbon dioxide on every exhale.

You should practice deep breathing throughout the day by inhaling deeply through your nose to fill your lungs with oxygen. Imagine that your lungs are a balloon that you need to fill to the max through inhaling. Take a deep breath and feel your diaphragm rise to its peak. Hold the expansion in your chest for a count of seven, then slowly begin to exhale as though you're letting the air out of the balloon. While exhaling, squeeze your abdominals from the top to the bottom extra hard and make a "sss" sound while releasing all the carbon dioxide. Push all the used-up air out of your lungs. The tight abdominal hold is a wonderful isometric exercise. Try performing this at least ten times daily. Mornings are probably most effective as your mind is clear of clutter from the day, and you can concentrate on the movements. On the other hand, doing this throughout the day is wonderful as it helps relieve the mental and emotional stress we all face.

TRANSFORMETRICS™ SECTION II
SPECIAL EXERCISES FOR SUPER JOINTS AND LIFELONG PAIN-FREE MOBILITY

*P*ain-free mobility is what we all hope to have for a lifetime. It always grieves me to see a person who is in obvious pain, whether it's a young man suffering with arthritis or an elderly woman with osteoporosis. And through my contacts at the gyms over the years and now through the Bronze Bow Publishing web site forum, I have met many people who have damaged and torn their muscles, joints, and ligaments. Many of the bodybuilders I know have overdone their weightlifting exercises to build body mass and paid a terrible price.

On our Bronze Bow Publishing web site forum we have several (proud to say) "ex" bodybuilders for whom *Transformetrics*™ has been a literal body saver. Through the following *Transformetrics*™ exercises, many of them have eliminated old injury pains and dramatically been helped to achieve strength beyond their imagination.

These exercises will stretch all the major muscle groups and lubricate all the major joints of your body. They can also help indicate where you are sore, weak, or stiff. If you feel pain while doing these exercises, listen to your body. It means you have a problem that requires immediate attention to correct. Lifelong injuries come when people try to push through pain. You may want to visit a chiropractor or sports doctor if you feel pain.

The simple warm-up moves on the following page only require a few minutes before your workout and can make an overall difference in your mobility down the road. All that is required is that you do seven repetitions of each movement. So practice them slowly and smoothly on a daily basis.

EXERCISE 1
NECK CIRCLES

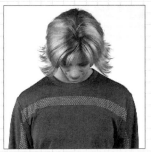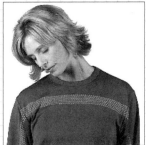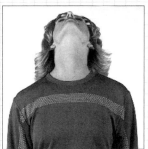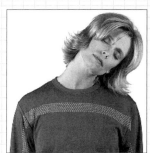

7 slow circles
in each direction.

EXERCISE 2
SHOULDER ROLLS

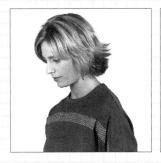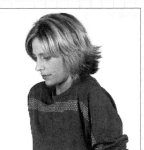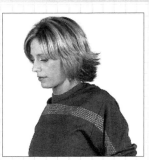

Raise shoulders up (toward ears),
back, and around. 7 slow reps.
Then up, forward, and around.

EXERCISE 3
ARM CIRCLES

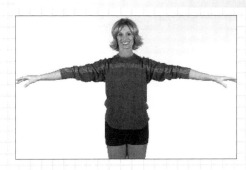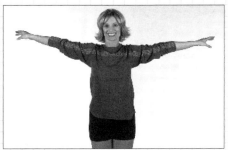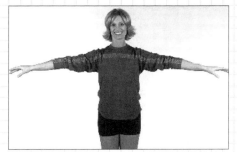

7 reps up, back, and around, then 7 reps up, forward, and around.

EXERCISE 4
TORSO TWIST

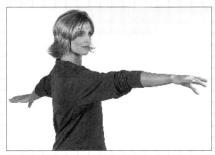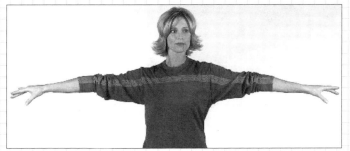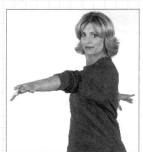

EXERCISE 5
TORSO ROTATION

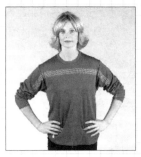 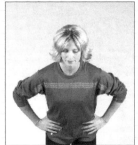 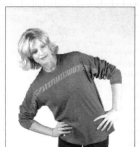 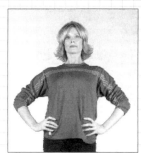 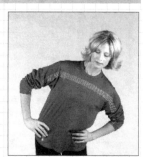

EXERCISE 6
HIP ROTATION

This is a circular motion.
7 reps each direction.

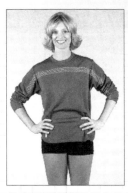 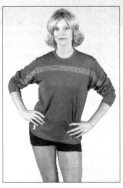 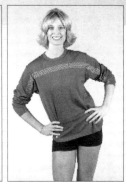 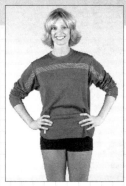

EXERCISE 7
WRIST ROTATION

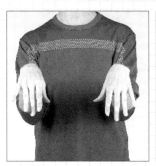 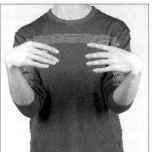 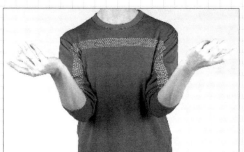 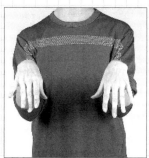

EXERCISE 8
HANDS AND FINGERS

Stretch and strengthen fingers and wrists by applying heavy tension and then relaxing.

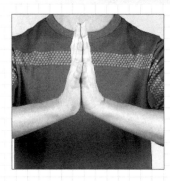 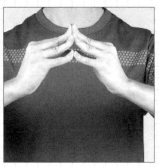 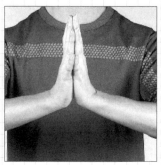

EXERCISE 9
ANKLE ROTATION

Rotate each ankle in each direction in small semi-circular movement. 7 reps and switch legs.

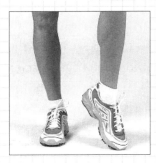 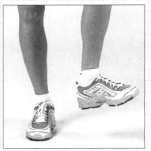 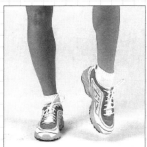

EXERCISE 10
TOE RAISE

Slowly raise up and down on toes. Just 7 reps is all that is neccessary.

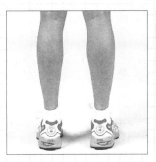 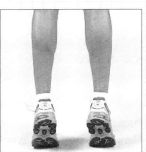

TRANSFORMETRICS™ SECTION III
FOUNDATIONAL EXERCISES FOR TOTAL STRENGTH AND DEVELOPMENT WITH SPECIAL EMPHASIS ON THE CHEST AND PECTORAL MUSCLES

"Walking is an excellent exercise. At 65, my grandmother began walking five miles a day. She's now 100—and we have no idea where she is."

—Robert B. Reich

Chest

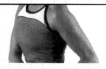

Most women are afraid to develop too much muscle in their chest area, thinking that they will lose the shape of their breasts and automatically turn into a female version of Tarzan. This can happen if you are lifting heavy weights and taking steroids, and the results are usually truly dreadful. But with the *Transformetrics*™ program, I almost feel as though I received a very inexpensive "boob job" or "breast enhancement" from a very expensive surgeon. With the DVR exercises and the push-ups as part of your routine, you will notice an amazing lift as muscle is being enhanced and/or created under our feminine chest. You will never look freakish while you use *Transformetrics*™.

As you progress with the exercises, you will start to feel the development of the muscle behind the fatty "female" tissue, which in turn causes the breasts to lift naturally. No pills, no surgery, just good old-fashioned push-ups and resistance training. I can't seem to get enough of the push-ups throughout the day. Co-workers have caught me on numerous occasions taking a break during the day and performing a quick set on the wooden boxes shown in the push-up section. I am amazed at how deep you can take these exercises and the numerous depths that are available due to the size of the boxes or stationary objects used during the push-ups.

Here's my promise: you will not be disappointed. Let's get to the exercises.

Please Note:

(DSR) means Dynamic Self-Resistance, where we actually put one set of muscles against another.

(DVR) refers to Dynamic Visualized Resistance, in which your imagination creates the tension in your muscles.

CH-1 (DSR)
LIEDERMAN CHEST PRESS

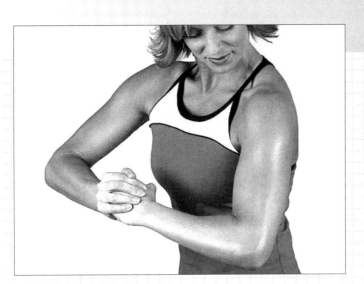

Clasp hands, or else grip them together as shown in photo. Keep them level with chest, then push one hand with the other back and forth across your chest just as far as you can each time. The harder you resist in this exercise, the more benefit you will get out of it. This exercise will outline your pectoral muscles better than any other movement, as it hits them direct.

CH-2 (DVR)
FULL RANGE PECTORAL CONTRACT

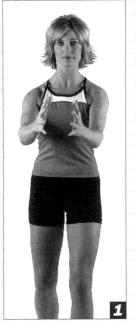
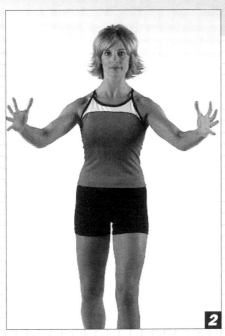
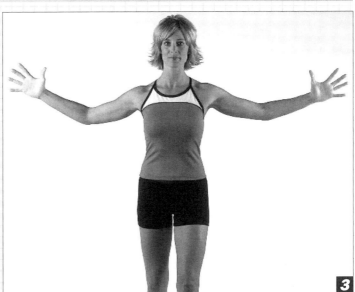

Stand with your left foot in front of your right foot and knee bent back straight (approximately one step, see photo). Hold hands in front, palms facing each other. Bring your hands back slowly with great tension until you feel your back muscles fully flexed. Hold for a count of one thousand one. Then move the hands slowly back to the original position while using great tension in your arms, shoulders, and pectoral muscles. Yes, the muscles will quiver.

CH-3 (DVR)
CROSSOVER PRESS DOWN

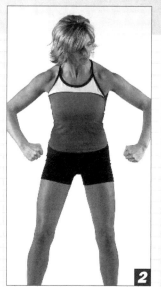
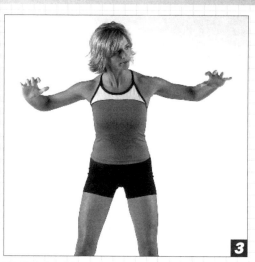
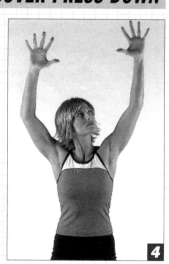

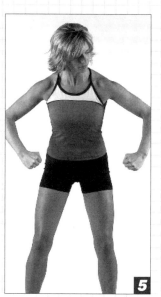
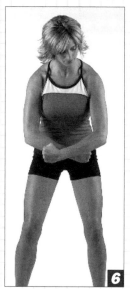

First, empty your lungs by crossing your arms in front of your chest and exhaling (see photo #1). Then raise your arms in a circular arc as though you are trying to reach the ceiling at both sides of the room while deeply inhaling. Slowly cross your arms in front with your right hand reaching left and your left hand reaching right. Powerfully contract the pectoral muscles as you try two or three times to reach farther while you exhale. Now raise your arms in a circular arc while inhaling.

This is both a powerful deep breathing and muscle contracting DVR exercise. It is a superb exercise to do anytime throughout the day to revitalize not only your musculature but also your brain with a fresh supply of oxygen. Do it often.

CH-4 (DVR)
ROPE PULL DOWN

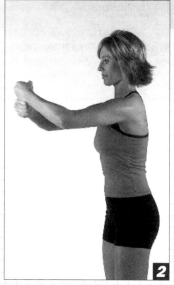
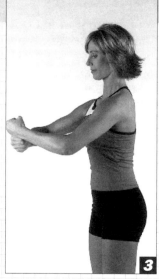

Begin with your hands placed around an imaginary rope just above head level (see photo #1). Left hand over right, start pulling down with your left hand against the strong resistance of your right hand. Make it hard and pull the full range of movement as shown. The key is the powerful contraction of the pectorals caused by the top and bottom hands resisting each other. Switch hands to right over left. Continue 3 to 5 times with each hand in the top position.

CH-5 (DSR)

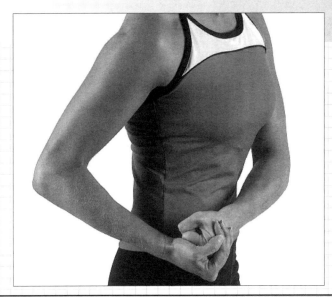

Place your left fist in the palm of your right hand on a level with the hips (see photo). Both hands are over your right hip with elbows bent. Against the powerful resistance of your right hand, endeavor to push your left hand down to the right side until your left elbow is no longer bent. This exercise is great for the pecs, arms, and shoulders.

CH-6 (DSR)
PULL APART, UP AND OVER

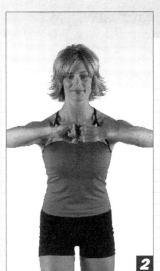
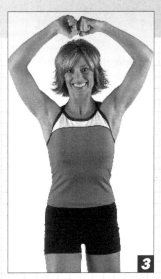

Grip the middle fingers of each hand as shown. Pull outward powerfully while raising your arms up, over, and back of your head. Maintain tension and reverse the direction of the arms until you reach the starting position. Continue 3 to 5 reps at extra heavy tension.

CH-7 (DSR)
LIEDERMAN PECTORAL CONTRACTION

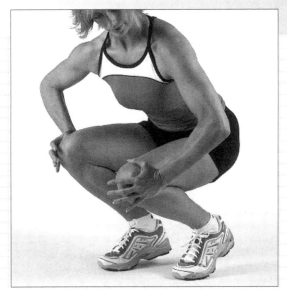

Initially, this may seem like an odd exercise, but wait till you try it. It is odd, but effective! Squat down as shown in the photo, heels approximately six inches apart and knees spread wide. Place your hands on the outside of your knees and endeavor to push your knees together against the powerful resistance of your knees pushing outward. Your pecs and arms get an incredible workout.

CH-8 (DSR)
C'MON AT YA!

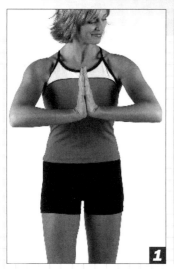 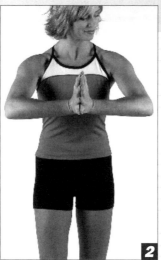 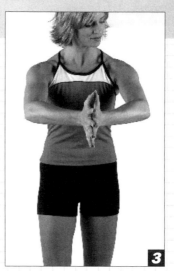

With your hands in a prayer posture at the center of your chest (see photo #1) and with both hands applying extra heavy resistance, slowly extend your arms. After achieving full extension, return to the start position while maintaining the tension. Each repetition will require 10 to 12 seconds to complete. 3 to 5 reps max, while maintaining extra-heavy tension.

CH-9 (DSR)

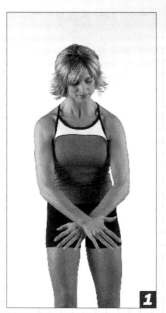 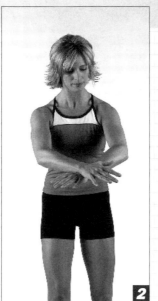 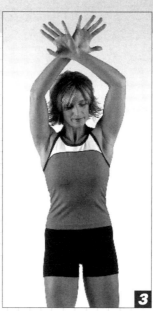

Assume the position shown in photo #1 with both your hands pressing powerfully toward each other. While maintaining this intense pressure with your arms bent, simultaneously inhale and slowly raise your hands to the position in photo #3. At the top of the movement, relax all your muscles momentarily while exhaling powerfully. Then regain the inward pressure of your hand and slowly lower to the starting position. Repeat the entire process 2 to 4 additional repetitions.

CH-10 (DVR)
(NOT PICTURED)

While standing erect, hands at sides, bear down on your shoulders and arms at the same time and consciously contract the pectoral muscles. This exercise is excellent for muscle control and can be practiced whenever you think of it throughout the day.

CH-11 (DSR)
(NOT PICTURED)

Stand with the palm of each hand pressing upon the top of your thighs. Your arms and legs are straight with all your muscles tightly contracted. Lean forward with great tension as your arms contract powerfully against your thighs and allow your hands to slide until they reach the knees. You'll notice that your abs as well as your pectorals and triceps can achieve peak contraction.

One More Thought...

In addition to the first 11 exercises presented so far, I encourage you to perform what I believe to be the four most important power calisthenic exercises in the entire realm of physical culture. They teach the muscles of the entire body to work together in unison and can dramatically enhance your speed, flexibility, balance, coordination, and endurance, in addition to the strength and aesthetics that are already achieved through performance of the first series of 11 exercises. These exercises in order of importance are in the next four pages to come:

1. The Furey Push-up

2. The Panther Stretch

3. The Atlas Push-up

4. The Furey Squat

THE FUREY PUSH-UP

In February 2003, when I injured my right shoulder, I first started with Panther Stretches during my healing process. This was prior to being able to perform the Furey Push-up in its entirety. Once I mastered the Panther Stretch and felt my shoulder heal in record time, I was able to have the flexibility and strength for the "swooping" action in the Furey Push-up. Now I have found amazing strength in my upper body partly due to these two exercises alone. Both of these exercises actually work every muscle from your neck to your toes.

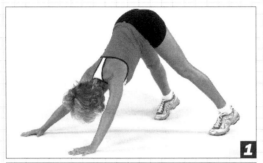

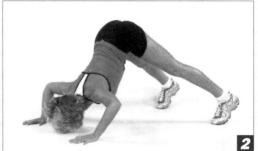

Photo #1. Start with your hands on the floor, shoulder-width apart, and your head tucked in and looking directly at your feet. Your feet are shoulder-width apart or slightly wider. Your legs and back are straight, and your butt is the highest point of the body.

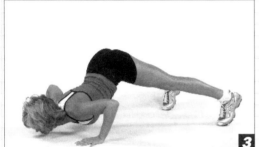

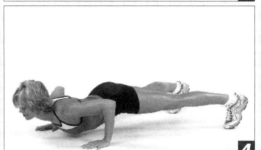

Photos #2-3-4-5. Bend your elbows while descending in a smooth circular arc almost brushing your chest and upper body to the floor as you continue the circular range of motion until your arms are straight, back flexed, and hips almost, but not quite, touching the floor.

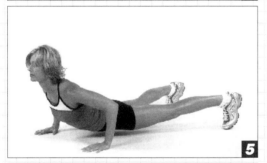

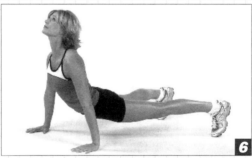

Photo #6. At the top of the movement, look at the ceiling while consciously flexing your triceps and exhaling.

Photo #7. Raise your hips and buttocks while simultaneously pushing back with straight arms, causing a complete articulation of both shoulder joints.

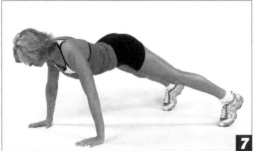

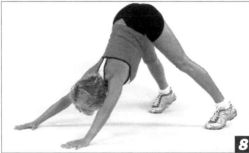

Photo #8. Arrive at the starting position with your legs and back straight, your head tucked in, and eyes looking at your feet.

Continue as smoothly and as fluidly as possible for as many repetitions as you can do.

At the beginning, anywhere from 15 to 25 repetitions is excellent. Once you can routinely do sets of 25 to 50 or more, you will have superb shoulder, chest, arm, and both upper and lower back development.

In my opinion this is the single greatest exercise. Repetition for repetition it delivers the highest level of strength, flexibility, and endurance of any calisthenic exercise known. In fact, it is the one exercise that comes closest to duplicating the exact movement of large jungle cats. It is truly one magnificent exercise.

THE PANTHER STRETCH

Start with your hands on the floor, shoulder-width apart, and your head tucked in and looking directly at your feet. Your feet are shoulder-width apart or slightly wider. Your legs and back are straight, and your butt is the highest point of the body as shown in Photo #1. Extend out into a semi-plank position, with a slight bend in the elbows as shown in Photo #2. At the top of the movement, look at the ceiling while consciously flexing your triceps and exhaling as shown in Photo #3. Return to starting position.

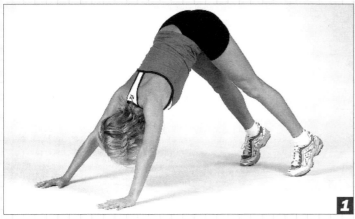

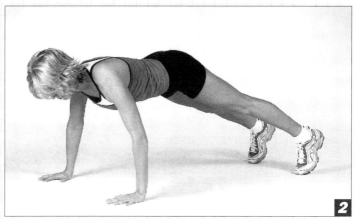

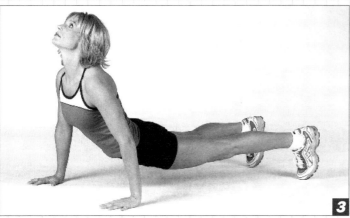

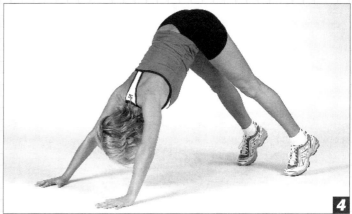

WE ARE ALL UNIQUE— BE *YOUR* OWN INDIVIDUAL

I encourage you to practice these exercises exclusively, including the two exercises on pages 48–49, and all the DVR exercises for the next three weeks. Please practice the nutritional advice and information on energy as well. They all work hand in hand.

After three weeks have passed, you will be able to listen to your body's needs as far as resistence, tempo, and sets and reps are concerned. You are your own best monitor, and only you can create the most effective program possible for results, knowing your mental, physical, and spiritual state. Do what feels best! You know yourself better than anyone else.

THE ATLAS PUSH-UP

I have been caught practicing these push-ups on numerous occasions at the office. I enjoy being able to get a deep stretch while performing the Atlas Push-ups and have noticed a difference in my overall strength thanks to the variation options.

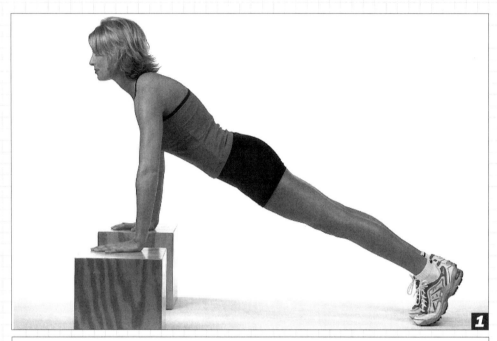

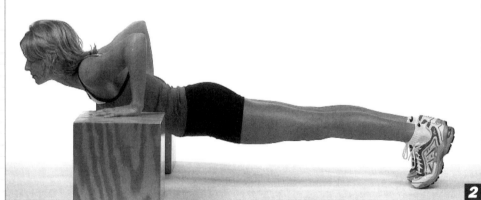

With two chairs side by side (between 18" and 26" apart, depending upon your shoulder width and arm length), place a hand on the seat of each chair (photo #1). Your body is extended in a sloping position with your feet on the floor. Now perform a push-up between the chairs, allowing your chest to descend as close to the floor as is comfortable (photo #2). Do not force yourself to descend beyond what is comfortable. In time your range of motion will naturally increase. Smoothly extend your arms to complete extension for one complete repetition.

Do as many as you can and as smoothly as possible. This is a superb deep breathing and pectoral development exercise. Atlas recommended that a total of 200 be performed if you want superb chest development. It is also a great exercise for the triceps of the upper arm and the latissimus dorsi muscles of the upper back. If you can perform sets of 25 or more, you are doing great.

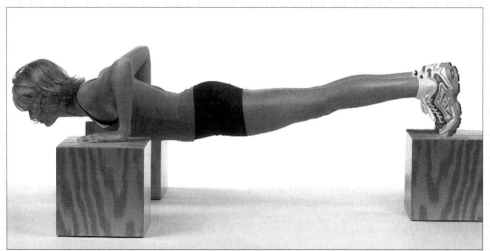

VARIATION

This exercise is performed exactly as above except that your feet are now elevated to a level equal to or higher than the hands. This variation changes the emphasis of development from the lower pectoral line to more of the middle pectoral muscles. If your feet are raised higher than the hands, the emphasis is changed to upper pectorals and deltoids. (please note: your abs get a great workout by maintaining flawless form as shown.)

THE FUREY SQUAT

This exercise is an amazing calisthenic. I do this exercise often, as it is a great cardiovascular move when done in high repetitions.

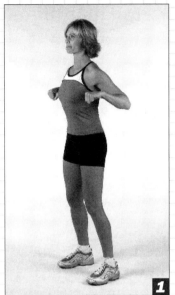 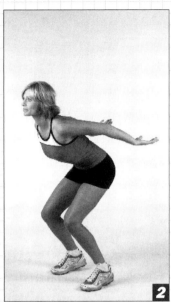 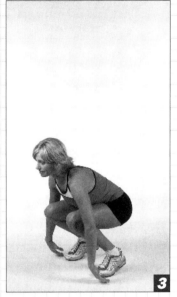

Photo #1. Feet approximately shoulder-width apart. Toes straight ahead. Hands in tight fists at shoulder level. Inhale deeply.

Photo #2. While keeping your back relatively straight (don't bend forward), bend your knees and descend to the bottom position.

Photo #3. Note the position of the hands reaching behind your back during the descent and brushing your knuckles on the ground at the bottom.

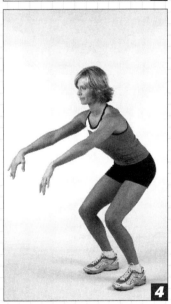 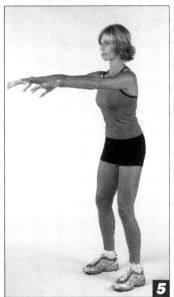 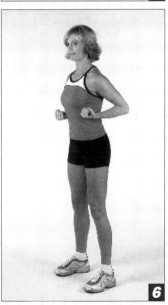

Photo #4. When you arrive at the bottom position, you will rise naturally to your toes. This is superb for your balance.

Photo #5. At this point your arms continue swinging forward and upward while simultaneously pushing off your toes and rising to the original standing position.

Photo #6. Your hands now form tight fists close to your sides at chest level. Inhale as you pull them in, exhale as you lower your body.

Repeat as smoothly and steadily as you can. Once you begin you'll notice that the arms take on a smooth, rhythmic motion similar to rowing a boat.

The entire movement of steps 1 to 6 is one continuous, smooth movement. 25 to 50 repetitions is a great start. 100 without stopping is excellent. Once you can do 350 or more in 20 minutes or less, you have accomplished the world's preeminent cardiovascular workout, not to mention a superb upper and lower leg workout. *Be careful. You may not be able to walk the next day!*

Question & Answer

Q: I have been hearing a lot about the dangers of hidden trans-fatty acids in the lunches served to children in school. What exactly are trans-fatty acids, and are they as bad as they say?

A: This is a huge problem across the nation. Trans-fatty acids are a result of hydrogenated fats, which are found in commercially packaged goods such as cookies, crackers, microwave popcorn, commercially fried foods such as French fries, as well as in vegetable shortening and some margarines. Indeed, any packaged goods that contain "partially-hydrogenated vegetable oils" or "shortening" probably contain trans-fats. And they are dangerous.

Since my mother retired from her government job, she decided to go back to work at a local elementary school lunchroom. She was amazed that the lunches served were loaded with hydrogenated fats and were mainly carbohydrate-related foods. The vegetable and fruit choices were minimal, if any. If you can send your child's lunch, *do!* There is an excellent book by Dr. Valerie Saxion called *Super Foods for Super Kids*. In her book Valerie offers simple, inexpensive, nutritious meals to pack for your child and all the basic nutritional information you need to introduce your child to a lifetime of vibrant health.

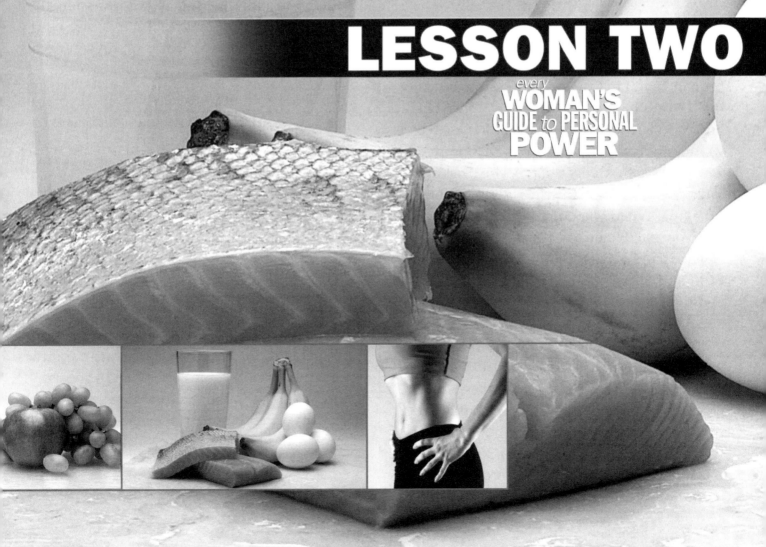

LESSON TWO

every
WOMAN'S
GUIDE *to* **PERSONAL**
POWER

Lesson Two: Nutrition

THE 80/20 DIET
(A Diet You Can Live With)

To create vibrant health and a toned shape you need to nourish your body with a balanced diet. Yes, it may require a lifestyle change. The old saying, "You are what you eat," holds true, and it's never too late to change your eating style. With every nutrient-dense food that you put in your mouth, your body thanks you by being able to reform itself from the inside and out. The energy derived from eating well is a gift all its own. I feel that most women are over-booked, over-stressed, over-tired, and we need all the natural nutrient assistance we can get!

One of my friends, Peter Arnold, is a prime example of "living again" by changing his eating style. He was supposed to meet my husband and I in Colorado last year to go skiing. I heard he had lost "a bunch" of weight, but wasn't sure what that meant. We were waiting for Peter at the base of Vail Mountain when this tall stranger approached me and said, "Hi, Wendie," with his arms reaching for a hug. When you don't recognize the person you once knew and only recognize the New Zealand accent, that defines "a bunch" of weight. I kept staring and saying, "Oh, my goodness, Peter, is that really you?" He said, "Yes, silly, it's me. How's my favorite Texas girl?" I couldn't get my lower jaw shut as I was in total shock. Peter had lost over 240 pounds—an entire person and then some! Come to find out he basically just started eating healthy as I'm going to describe for you in this chapter. He used the 80/20 rule and made it his lifestyle. I am very proud of him

and his accomplishments and know that he continues to work out and be active as well as eat healthy.

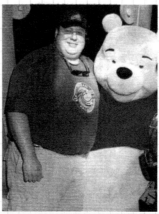 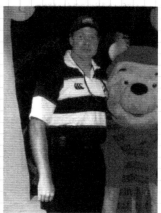

Peter Arnold: Before, 2002   Peter Arnold: After, 2003

Will this approach work for the average American and lead you to health, strength, and rejuvenation? *Absolutely!* You do not need to be on a fad diet to become fit. All you need is a healthy one.

Growing up in Texas our typical meal would consist of fried chicken, fried okra, French fries, and maybe some corn. Obviously, that's not going to fuel your body for peak performance. Fortunately, my father always had a garden and would bring a plate of fresh vegetables to every meal, or I don't think I would have ever learned about "real food." In high school I made the lifestyle change and educated myself on how to eat healthy in a fast-food-joint-on-every-corner world. I found that I was less stressed, less tired, had healthier skin, and my grades improved beyond my parent's belief. I no longer put projects and papers off until the last minute due to exhaustion and lack of concentration, which made a big difference. A healthy diet has now helped assist me in my current phase of life by offering 100 percent of the energy I need for my family, friends, and career. It feels great!

Why Do We Get Fat?

Here's the "skinny" on fat. Everything we consume contains energy or calories. If we do not burn the calories that we consume, they get stored as body fat. Obviously, the more calories consumed versus burned equals the fatter we get. Women usually refer to fat terms such as "pinching more than an inch," "cottage cheese," "rolly-polly," and "thunder thighs." If you think or feel that any of these horrible catty terms apply to you, don't worry. You will be able to shed the weight and ditch the tag names for good. It just won't be overnight. Rome wasn't built in a day, and neither will your goal for building your perfect temple.

The true healthy way to lose weight and keep it off is to approach your new eating style slowly and calmly. While training with *Transformetrics*™ and eating healthy, you will begin to see the lithe muscles that have been in hibernation for so long. And you will look and feel younger. It is a fact that overeating is the major cause of premature aging. Most people who overeat are undernourished, and overeating becomes a compulsory habit and develops what is known as "artificial appetite." It ends up exhausting the body's ability to cope. Scientific research has proven that when a nourishing diet is eaten sparingly, aging can be delayed and you can add years of vitality to your life.

Tips for Obese Women. Read Dr. Valerie Saxion's book, *How to Stop Candida and Other Yeast Infections in Their Tracts*. Over 90 percent of the U.S. population have some degree of Candida overgrowth in their bodies. Getting rid of this problem could be your first step to losing weight effectively along with my rec-

ommended meal planning. Also, Valerie Saxion's book, *How to Feel Great All the Time*, details the importance of detoxifying the body, which is another key to living right and shedding pounds. One of my favorite detoxifying methods is Valerie's "Creation's GI Cleanse and Detox." It helped cleanse, energize, and refresh my mind and body and, believe it or not, my spirit. Once I was rid of the toxins in my body, my spirit thanked me in many ways. Many women suffer from depression, and detoxifying, exercising, and eating right can make a major difference. Pills do not have to be your answer.

Where to Start

First, memorize these facts:

3,500—number of calories stored in one pound of fat.

35—number of calories burned by one pound of muscle each day.

2—number of calories burned by one pound of fat each day.

Do the simple math with me. If you add 10 pounds of muscle to your physique through *Transformetrics*™ while maintaining your present weight, your body will burn off 1 pound of body fat every 10 days (350 calories per day X 10 days = 3,500 calories). That's naturally. If you restrict your caloric intake by approximately 500 calories a day, you could lose 1 pound of fat every 5 days. In 90 days that equates to 18 pounds of body fat that has now been replaced with sculpted muscle. You will notice an extreme change in the way your body looks and feels not to mention the new way your clothes begin to fit.

Once this starts to happen, I give you permission to start your shopping spree for your new wardrobe! Oops. Maybe I better back pedal or spouses will be upset with me. So, I will just say to use your best judgment and do something nice for yourself as a reward throughout each goal that you achieve. Motivation always helps to succeed. Unfortunately for my husband, shopping motivates me!

Food Facts

Fat, protein, and carbohydrates represent the three major food groups. A healthy diet for maximum weight loss consists of 15 percent fat, 15 percent protein, and 70 percent unrefined carbohydrates. Once you reach a point where you are as fat free as you want to be, you will slowly add both protein and fat to your diet and rely less on carbohydrates, or you will keep losing weight. I just want to maintain my weight now so my diet consists of 25 percent fat, 35 percent protein, and 50 percent carbohydrates. Using this scale of percentages I stay within an average weight of 120 to 125 pounds, which is where I want to be.

Remember, everyone is unique and will require different percentages for these three groups to work in their favor. Experiment and record your changes. You should use *The Power Living Journal* to help you log the quantities of each group so you can see if something needs adjusting. To define the three groups in more detail, let's look at each one separately.

Fat

You guessed it—if you eat fatty foods, you get fat! While eating a small amount of fat is essential for your body to function, too much will not only increase the size of your trouble zones but increase your risk for heart disease, cancer, and diabetes.

Fat is found in everything, even fruit. An average apple has 1 gram of fat. Choose the sources of your fat intake wisely and try to stay away from most saturated and trans-fats. These are found in margarine, fatty meats, milk, cheese, and some plant foods that include coconut and palm oil. Some "bad fats" that you should steer away from are produced foods, such as pastries, deep fried fast foods, potato chips, and confectionery.

Protein

Protein is one of the basic components of food and makes all life possible. Amino acids are the building blocks for proteins. Antibodies, enzymes, and hormones are proteins. Proteins provide for the transport of nutrients, oxygen, waste, and other factors throughout the body.

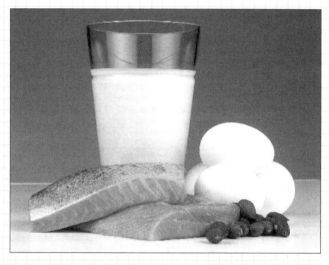

I am a big advocate of protein as it is a key ingredient in a balanced diet and helps to build and repair muscle. Like anything else, too much isn't a good thing. Protein will be stored as fat if you overdo your intake. You need to choose the best sources of lean protein as most protein is found in foods that are high in fat.

There's plenty of buzz on soy and whey protein in health and fitness articles as well as programs on television. There are many different types of proteins out there that even include vegetable, rice, egg, casein, and hemp. I am going to touch base on the two most popular—soy and whey.

Whey protein: Seems to be popular more for men, but anyone can consume this protein. There is a huge myth that soy protein will give a guy "man boobs." Anyone can take soy or whey. I usually stick with soy because as women we need the added benefits it offers for our complex makeup. Whey protein is a byproduct of cheese making, which yields a natural, high purity protein product without any added preservatives. Whey helps maintain adequate glutathione levels to aid the immune system and increase muscle stamina. During times of stress, such as exercise, the glutathione levels decrease, and whey will replenish these if taken within two hours before or after exercise activity. Whey also has been proven to increase fat loss and muscle gain in comparison to eating healthy, balanced meals alone.

Soy protein: A significant number of research studies support claims that soy consumption can help you lose weight. Combined with my exercise plan, it makes a powerful combination for weight loss. While there is no "magic bullet" for weight loss, healthy nutritional choices are vital to any weight-loss plan. Recent studies show that soy protein is a low-fat source of high-quality protein (compared to many other protein sources). Soy protein helps reduce the hunger cravings we all fight. Because soy is a low-glycemic index food, you won't experience dramatic peaks and valleys in blood sugar levels. This minimizes insulin secretion and subsequent fat storage (insulin stores the extra sugar in your bloodstream as fat). Soy is also a good source of energy from the protein. We all need extra energy to work out!

I've found a delicious line of soy products that I use personally. Perhaps you've tasted some really bad soy products in the past, but Revival is delicious (it doesn't taste like soy). I eat one bar or shake each day to give me the boost I need. Some soy products have a chalky texture whereas this one does not. It's so easy to blend and only takes a matter of seconds in the Revival shaker. I enjoy the fact that I can dump in a Revival soy packet, add water, shake, and go. It's easier than making a bowl of cereal and much better for you.

Just one Revival shake or bar contains the amount of soy isoflavones found in 6 cups of soymilk as well as 16 to 20 grams of soy protein. They also have great-tasting soy chips that will help you avoid unhealthy snacks. Revival is the #1 doctor-recommended soy protein supplement because of great taste, fast results, medical research, and patented benefits.

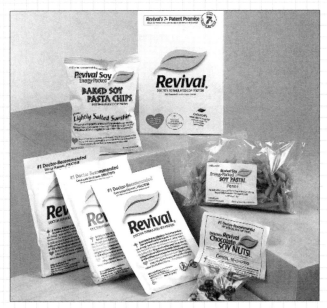

Combined with a proper diet and *Transformetrics*™, Revival is a powerful tool to help you control your weight and boost your energy. To order or find out more information, call 1-800-REVIVAL or go online to www.revivalsoy.com. Use REFERENCE NUMBER 3756 to receive a free variety pack with your first 30-day shake or bar purchase. Tell them I sent you!

Carbohydrates

Carbohydrates are the "quick energy" fuel suppliers for the body and the mind. They come from the starchy part of plant foods and easily convert to sugar in the body. Therefore, these foods are burned at a fast rate for energy. The broken down form of carbohydrates is known as a form of sugar called glucose. A certain amount is stored in the liver as an energy reserve when it's needed by the body. To a lesser degree, glycogen is stored in the muscles as a key fuel source, especially during exercise. Keep in mind, if they are not used, they are poorly stored and converted to fat.

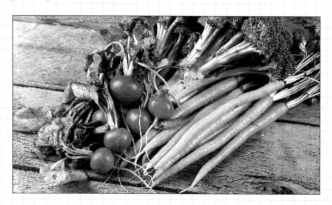

There are simple and complex carbohydrates found in this category. Simple carbohydrates come in good forms, such as those found in fruits of all types, and bad forms, such as those found in all sugars. You should keep the level of bad simple carbohydrates to a minimum. If you don't, you won't reach your goal due to the concentrated sugars. These "bad carbs" can cause blood sugar levels to change more rapidly than normal, allowing swings in sugar levels that can cause symptoms such as fatigue, irritability, and appetite increases.

Complex carbohydrates form the basis of a healthy balanced diet. They include all vegetables, whole-grain breads and cereals, rice and pasta. Soy protein contains complex carbohydrates that are slowly metabolized and do not

cause a rapid rise in blood glucose levels or over-secretion of insulin, thus decreasing fat storage. If you are trying to lose or maintain your weight, try not to eat many carbohydrates after four o'clock. That way you still have the remainder of the day to burn up what has been stored before they sneak to your trouble zone like a thief in the night.

How Much of Each Group Should You Eat?

With a goal to lose body fat quickly and safely, my food plan is designed for eating 15 percent fat, 15 percent protein, and 70 percent carbohydrates. All you will have to worry about is keeping your daily fat grams between 20 to 25 if you are a woman and between 30 to 40 grams for a man. Of course, the fewer fat grams you consume, the quicker the fat is lost. But do not go lower than 10 percent of your daily caloric intake or your body won't be able to fabricate hormones needed for good health, and you will feel hungry and edgy all the time.

It's best to try and eat five to six small meals daily. I call it grazing. This keeps your metabolism on call all day and helps to maintain your weight.

Water, water, and more water should be consumed on a daily basis. It is recommended to drink 8 to 12 eight-ounce glasses daily, and increase the amount when conducting more physical fitness than normal. If you are a soda addict and not big on aqua, try replacing the habit with flavored water until you get used to the pure thing. You will be amazed at how much weight can be lost through increasing water alone, not to mention its benefits to the skin and the energy it triggers.

"To deny your body is to be a no-body."

A Balanced Diet

A balanced diet should contain the following:

2–3 servings of low-fat dairy products

2–3 servings of lean protein

3–5 servings of vegetables

2–4 servings of fruit

6–12 servings of whole-grain breads, grains, pastas, rice, or cereal

This guideline was formulated to fit this low-fat weight-loss plan. I have made adjustments so that the maximum amount of body fat can be lost and yet ensure optimal health and nutrition. In the following paragraphs you will be advised of which foods are recommended for the low-fat eating plan and how much of these foods constitutes a serving. There will be three different lists to choose from, and you may switch what you eat daily as often as you would like, as long as it's on the list. All you need to do is just make sure you are still attaining the servings listed above.

Let's look closer at each specific food group and determine what establishes a practical serving in each of the five (actually six) distinctive food groups. You know the ones—you learned them in kindergarten.

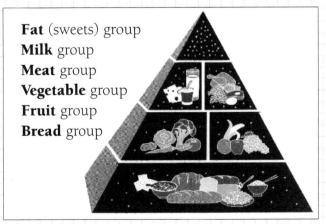

Fat (sweets) group
Milk group
Meat group
Vegetable group
Fruit group
Bread group

Eat 6 to 11 Servings of Limited Complex Carbohydrates (preferably natural and whole-grain varieties)

Note: Typically speaking, depending on your size, men will eat the amount closer to the maximum number of servings, and women will eat closer to the minimum. However, women who are more than 20 pounds overweight may opt for the maximum amount.

Complex carbohydrates provide high energy and generally include whole-grain breads and cereals, rice, pasta, and all grains, plus a variety of high carbohydrate vegetables.

List One

One serving is equal to:
2 slices of whole wheat bread
1/2 bagel
1 English muffin
3 cups of air-popped popcorn
1/2 cup hot cooked cereal
3/4 cup dry cold cereal
2/3 cup cooked pasta or rice
1/3 cup barley
1 ounce of pretzels
8 low fat medium crackers
4 rice cakes
1 medium potato
1 small yam or sweet potato
1 cup beets or peas
1 cup of corn
1 large corn on the cob
3/4 cup Jerusalem artichoke
1 cup acorn squash

Let's look at the maximum allowance first for men and for women who are 20 pounds or more overweight. On an average day a sample of what you could eat from this list is as follows: A whole bagel for breakfast (2 servings), 1-1/2 cups of rice with lunch (2 servings), a generous amount of pretzels for a snack (2 servings), 2 cups of pasta for dinner (3 servings), and 2 rice cakes for snack (1/2 serving), and still be within the fat-loss range.

Keep in mind: You still need to pick servings from the next two lists as well. If it is starting to already sound like too much food, then you may go closer to the minimum if you want, or anywhere in between, and still be within the range of healthy eating.

Eat 6 or More Servings of Vegetables (preferably much more of these complex carbohydrates)

Note: Any of these vegetables except those on the previous list is considered to be fair game.

List Two

One serving is equal to (1/2 cup cooked or 1 cup raw):

- Asparagus
- Broccoli
- Brussel sprouts
- Cabbage
- Carrots
- Cauliflower
- Celery
- Chicory
- Collard greens
- Cucumber
- Eggplant
- Endive
- Escarole
- Frozen mixed vegetables
- Green or yellow beans
- Kale
- Leeks
- Lettuce
- Mushrooms
- Okra
- Onions
- Parsnips
- Peppers
- Radishes
- Rutabagas
- Shallots
- Sprouts
- Squash

In addition to what I recommended you could eat from List One, you can have six or more servings from List Two. If anyone feels hungry after eating the recommended servings from each list, I think you better give me a call and we should chat. You can eat over six whole cups of vegetables throughout your day along with the servings from List One and *still* lose weight! Why? Because vegetables are *very* low in calories and at the same time are filling. You can never eat enough vegetables—at least that's what my father used to always tell me. Actually, I doubt that the average person actually eats enough out of this category so make this one a conscious effort!

Vegetables not only help to keep you looking good, but the nutrients in them ward off all kinds of illnesses and diseases. I even have my son, Keegan, hooked on the vegetable message. Of course, since he is three, I have him convinced that "Popeye muscles" will appear after each and every bite. If I need to tell you the same, then I will! You will learn to love them if you don't already. I have my favorites, but I always try to add new vegetables to my diet. If a little garlic or seasoning helps you down a certain veggie, fine with me! It's not going to diminish the nutrients one bit to add a little "spice" to your life.

Eat 2 to 4 Servings of Simple Carbohydrates Daily—Fruit

One serving equals:

1 large piece of any fruit: apple, orange, pear, etc.

1 cup berries of any kind

1 cup mango or papaya

1-1/2 cups of strawberries or watermelon

1/2 cantaloupe, grapefruit, or large plantain

1/4 honeydew melon or pineapple

1 large banana

20 cherries

20 grapes

4 persimmons or kumquats

3 large plums or tangerines

Wow! Is this crazy or what? More food! Two servings of any combination above and you can still lose body fat.

Eat 2 to 3 Servings of Lean Protein

One serving equates to 4 to 6 ounces of white chicken, turkey, or fish. Keep in mind that all poultry should be cooked without the skin and without fat.

List Three
Protein/Fat

Poultry (4 ounces cooked)

	Protein Grams	Fat Grams
Turkey Breast	34	1
Turkey Drumstick	33	4.5
Turkey Thigh	31	5
Chicken Breast	35	4.5
Chicken Drumstick	37	6.8
Chicken Thigh	31	5

Fish (4 ounces cooked)

	Protein Grams	Fat Grams
Mahi Mahi	20.8	.8
Haddock	23	1
Cod	26	1
Abalone	16	1
Sole	19	1
Pike	25	1
Scallops	26	1
Tuna in water	34	1
Squid	20	1.8
Flounder	34	2.3
Red Snapper	26	2.3
Sea Bass	25	3.4
Halibut	31	4
Trout	30	4

Vegetarian Sources

3 Egg Whites	9	1
1/2 Cup Beans	9	1
1/2 Cup Soft Tofu	10	6
1/2 Cup Firm Tofu	10	11

On the following list, fat grams and protein grams are listed next to each protein/fat source. Please note: multiply both protein grams and fat by 1.5 if you use 6-ounce portions as recommended.

Once you have reached your fat loss goal, you may switch your levels of protein, fat, and carbohydrate percentages to a higher amount and still gain zero body fat. It is up to you to monitor your intake from all three lists and review at what point your body starts storing fat, then adjust again accordingly.

Eat 2 to 3 Dairy Foods Daily

One serving equals	Protein Grams	Fat Grams
8 ounces low-fat yogurt	12	4
8 ounces no-fat yogurt	12	0
8 ounces 1% milk	9	3
8 ounces skim milk	9	0
4 ounces 1% cottage cheese	14	1
2 tablespoons no-fat cream cheese	2	0
2 slices no-fat cheese	12	0
1/2 cup no-fat ice cream	2	0

If you are lactose intolerant, I recommend Revival Soy Products. Just be aware of your fat grams.

Review to Lose Body Fat on the "Hurry Up"

1. **EAT YOUR MINIMUM FOR THE DAY.**

   - 6 to an unlimited number of servings of vegetables (both raw and cooked)

   - 6–11 servings of complex carbohydrates

   - 2–4 servings of fruit (fresh, frozen, or canned in juice with no sugar)

   - 2–3 servings of lean protein, 4-6 ounces each

   - 2–3 servings of dairy or substitute dairy products

2. **EAT OFTEN.** Ideally, graze 5 to 6 times a day, waiting no more than 4 hours without eating.

3. **HYDRATE YOURSELF.** I cannot stress this enough! Drink lots of pure water, 8 to 12 eight-ounce glasses each day. I always carry a water bottle with me everywhere I go. Water helps every single part of your body function with ease. If you drink coffee or alcohol at any level, it makes it hard to hydrate yourself. They are both diuretics and flush fluids from the body.

4. **HAVE FUN.** It's acceptable to enjoy yourself from time to time. Matter of fact, I recommend it! Eating something special out of the blue is okay. Whether it is a sweet or just something downright fattening, your body actually craves this from time to time. If you don't allow yourself a reward once in a while, you will not be able to have a successful eating lifestyle. Cut yourself some slack because you have worked hard to get to where you are! One bite of cake isn't going to kill you. But you don't have to eat the entire piece either.

5. **DON'T OVERDO IT.** Be good to yourself and listen to your body. Every individual is completely different. Maybe you are doing this program with a friend or spouse (I encourage this, by the way), and you may have similar goals, but you will get there in your own particular way.

6. **BE SMART.** Remember, everything in moderation. Once you are on the road to success, you will see it immediately and so will others. Maintain what you were doing. There's no need to go to extremes. Before you know it, your friends and family will want to know your secret. (Always share.)

These guidelines will get you moving in the right direction and help you achieve your goal. Keep in mind the importance of adding more protein to your diet and cutting down on your carbohydrates. You don't want to lose too much weight, meaning muscle weight. I wouldn't want all of your hard *Transformetrics*™ work to go down the tubes.

"Honoring your body as the sacred temple for the divine within you and the physical self is the only way to be energized and healthy enough to accomplish God's will for your life."

Is Transformetrics™ the Only Form of Exercise I Practice?

No, but I do some form of *Transformetrics*™ daily. Some days it is all I do, and it's very intense. Other days are a bit lighter, such as when I dance or run. It has been interesting that *Transformetrics*™ seemed to bring me back to my dancing roots. Little did I realize, but I have actually been doing *Transformetrics*™ types of movements all my life. The way I concentrate and contract certain muscles to plie or arabesque in dance class is basically the same as I do with *Transformetrics*™.

"Being powerful is like being a lady. If you have to tell people you are, you aren't."
—Margaret Thatcher

LESSON THREE

every
WOMAN'S
GUIDE *to* **PERSONAL**
POWER

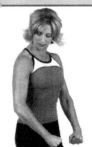 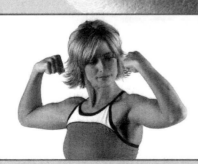 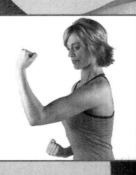 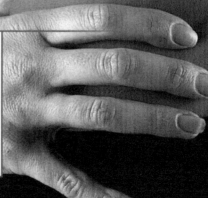

Lesson Three
AN INTRODUCTORY PROGRAM FOR THE WEAK AND OBESE

Most of us burn the candle at both ends, and the common complaint I hear when I'm calling on business clients is that people are "running on empty," "exhausted," "rundown," and an occasional person is "sleep walking." Since I gave birth to my son and often find myself having to perform with precious little sleep, I know what that complaint is all about.

But I am also acutely aware that there are hundreds of thousands of people who for numerous reasons look at a program such as *Transformetrics*™, shake their heads, and walk away because they feel they don't even have the energy to begin it. It might be related to the exhausting, debilitating effects of obesity or from a prolonged lack of physical activity or a prolonged illness or from depression. They realize that getting in shape is tremendously important, but it just seems too overwhelming.

So how do we get more energy to even start? With so much of our personal success related to our energy level, it's a real concern. If you are dragging through your days, it's going to take its toll on your financial, emotional, social, intellectual, and spiritual success in life. And if the cause is related to the effects of obesity, it can be life-threatening to not take action.

Many people look to boost their energy level through vitamins, energy drinks, and a wide variety of ideas and gimmicks that saturate the market. The truth is that most "energy boosting" products are not healthy for you—read the labels and you'll see the problems. Certainly, we need to take vitamins and consume the right nutrients daily through our food intake, but what else should we be doing to get our bodies, minds, and spirits revitalized?

I'd like to introduce you to a Dynamic Visualized Resistance (DVR) Exercise Program that John Peterson developed for people who need special help to get in good enough shape to begin the *Transformetrics*™ *Training System*. It is a marvelous way to slowly develop the muscles of your entire body and restore your energy levels.

> *"You cannot expect to expend the same amount of energy to get out of a problem as you did to get into it."*—Albert Einstein

Take Control of Your Life

Whether you are obese, weak, exhausted, depressed, or lacking self-confidence, you can begin to take back control of your life at this very moment. Whether you feel like it or not, the Bible says that you are "fearfully and wonderfully made" (Psalm 139:14). Within you, however silent or damaged it may have become, is the person created in the image of God whom God desires to strengthen and create a new future for. Your life is your life, and by God's grace and help you can turn things around.

If you are obese or weak, you were probably never taught the fundamental principles of good nutrition and exercise. For you, the first step toward a renewal of energy and change in your life is to implement the balanced diet that I laid out in the previous chapter. *It's time to break the mold on your diet and give your body a chance to renew itself!* Make that the one goal that you focus on and accomplish within the next month. Besides the changes you'll feel in your body, your creative power will begin to surge. You will feel energized intellectually, emotionally, and physically. It is within your reach, and *you can do it!*

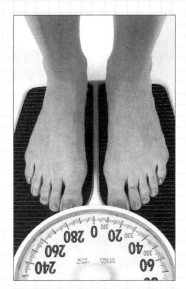

Next, you need to be true and honest with yourself in every aspect of your life. Refuse to hide behind your reflection any longer. It's time to face your fears, frustrations, and desires. Don't hold back. This is not about blame. It's about identifying the truth and taking *responsibility*. Responsibility means to empower yourself to *respond with ability*. I realize this takes courage, but I guarantee there is a way out of whatever situation you find yourself stuck in.

Stop letting guilt get the best of you. If there is true guilt in your life from past sins or from failing to obey what you know God has said, bring it to him and be forgiven. Don't let it keep you trapped. "If we confess our sins, he is faithful and just and will forgive us our sins and purify us from all unrighteousness" (1 John 1:9). God can cleanse away the guilt of sin instantly by the blood of Jesus (1 John 1:7).

If there are fears or other things that are holding you back, take these to God in prayer. "Do not be anxious about *anything*, but in everything, by prayer and petition, with thanksgiving, present your requests to God. And the peace of God, which transcends all understanding, will guard your hearts and minds in Christ Jesus" (Philippians 4:6–7). Nothing is outside the scope of prayer and God's care.

And nothing in the universe is stronger than the peace of God to bring order and rest to our troubled minds and hearts.

Opening the door to a renewed relationship with God will make a huge impact on your life and outlook. He will not allow you to focus on the bad things that have happened to you in the past. He will direct your focus to the joy He has for you today and for the positive things He wants for your life. Positive things such as:

- A beautiful, healthy body that is pleasing to you.

- A keen, clear mind that allows you to discover solutions to every challenge you face in life.

- A job or career that you find fulfilling.

- A wonderful relationship with the mate of your dreams.

- A solid spiritual foundation that brings meaning and purpose to every facet of your life as well as the confidence that you never again have to face anything alone because God is with you.

Finally, brethren, whatever things are true, whatever things are noble, whatever things are just, whatever things are pure, whatever things are lovely, whatever things are of good report, if there is any virtue and if there is anything praiseworthy, meditate on these things.
—Philippians 4:8

The Power of Being Positive

The key to creating the life you want begins when you clearly identify your goals. The more vivid and specific the details of your goals, the better the results. The master key, however, is to identify your desires and to put it down on paper so that it is transformed from the realm of thought to the realm of action.

First, take out a pen and notepad and make a list of the priority issues you don't want in your life. If you don't want to be overweight, for instance, it's essential that you write it down. Or if you don't want to be weak or to have back pain or to be the brunt of someone's jokes—you get the idea. It's not hard, but it's *essential* that you document it.

Okay, now flip the notepad sheet and write down anything that you sincerely want. While it doesn't have to all be fitness related, be specific about fitness-related goals that you want to accomplish. For instance, if you are obese and desire to lose 150 pounds, document it as a goal you're going to achieve.

The next action step is focus on one fitness-related goal and make a short-term goal that is within your reach. Make it a goal you can accomplish within the next month. Perhaps it is to implement the new diet and bring your eating habits under control. Perhaps it is to lose 10 pounds. If it is attainable, you will be encouraged to lose the rest of your weight once you see that you can accomplish this goal first. By taking steps of responsibility for your life, you know that it's in your hands to go all the way!

In order for you to have abundance in all areas of life, in order to move up to a superior level of life, your mind, body, and spirit must all start moving in the same direction. When that happens, "miracles" begin to happen. If you surround yourself with positive reinforcement in what you see, hear, think, and verbalize, and if you follow through with positive action—you will meet with a positive outcome. It is inevitable!

An Exercise Program for the Weak and Obese

It's time to give you a specific program of exercise that will sculpt, strengthen, and reshape your body without putting your joints, tendons, ligaments, bones, and muscles in danger of injury. To accomplish this we will use Dynamic Visualized Resistance Exercises (DVR) combined with the right aerobic exercises to totally transform your physique. Although I explained the method in Lesson One, let's take a few minutes to review it.

As stated previously, many exercise systems can harm the body, and this is especially true for people who are overweight or very weak. Exercise machines and free weights can literally tear muscles, wear out joints, tendons, and ligaments, and damage the vascular system. Jogging, long distance running, and high intensity aerobics can injure bones in the feet, legs, and lower back as well as expend great energy needlessly.

The DVR system is nothing more than stretching (extending and contracting) with great tension. If you watch a lion at the zoo or a household cat, this stretching takes only a few seconds and is done many times throughout the day. You'll notice that it stretches its entire body with great tension. The tension is so powerful it actually builds muscles. The inner resistances produced by the tension builds muscle fibers just as much as any form of external resistance whether by weights or machines. *But* since the resistance is perfectly controlled throughout the entire range of motion, no physical harm is done.

Translate these gentle movements to an exercise system and you *energize* the body. And best of all, these exercises require no gym and no equipment. They can be done anywhere and at any time regardless of your size or shape. In fact, they are the *perfect* exercise system in and of themselves.

To get the most benefit from this program keep the following information in mind:

- **AEROBICS.** This DVR Exercise Program will develop your entire body. But I also recommend that you try to walk at least 30 minutes each day if you want to lose body fat. Swimming is also a great addition. I don't recommend running or jogging until you are in good shape.

- **FREQUENCY.** DVR exercises should be done daily. At first you should use relatively light tension that allows you to complete 10 to 12 repetitions per set before the muscles feel fatigued. At that point go immediately to the next exercise and progress through the entire series of 12 exercises, doing 10 to 12 repetitions each. Then repeat the entire circuit of 12 exercises at least once but preferably twice. Once you have mastered the movements you can apply greater tension. Your sets and repetitions will then change to reflect the following:

REPETITIONS		SETS
MODERATE	8-10	3 max
HEAVY	6-8	2-3 max
VERY HEAVY	3-5	2 max

- **TENSION.** The key to the system is the amount of tension used. When you are starting out, vary the amount of *tension* until it feels comfortable. If you use only a small amount of *tension,* you will maintain muscle tone but not build muscle. Too much tension can strain tendons and ligaments and even cause headaches. The right amount will develop the muscle fibers every bit as much as weights or machines but without the debilitating effects. So follow the guideline and realize that these exercises can be every bit as taxing as weightlifting. A word to the wise: Don't overdo it.

- **BREATHING.** DVR exercises should be performed slowly and with great tension while breathing deeply. Breathe using both nose and mouth. Inhale on the way back (or up). Exhale on the way forward (or down). Between exercises practice power breathing from Lesson One.

Muscle Size and Strength

Working out with DVR will require 20 to 25 minutes for a complete workout of 3 sets of 10 reps of each exercise. It can result in a dramatic increase in muscle size and strength as well as develop a sense of body awareness that allows you to contract any and every muscle group in your entire body at will. If after you have regained your strength you want to add other exercises, feel free to do so and take your development to the epitome of strength and athletic development. Good luck, and please send me photos to let me see what you accomplish. In future editions of this book, I would like to have some of my best students model for the photos. I hope you will be one of them.

The DVR Routine

1. Neck Roll

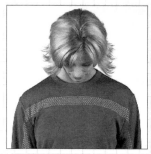 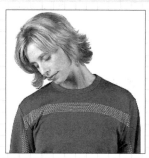 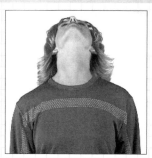 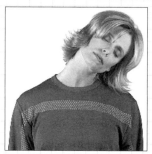

Stand with your feet side by side, hands at your side, and slowly roll your head to the right while contracting the muscles in your neck. Circle all the way around for one repetition. Continue until you have completed 10 reps. Then reverse direction and complete 10 more while circling to the left. Start with light tension and gradually build.

2. Atlas Biceps Flex and Press

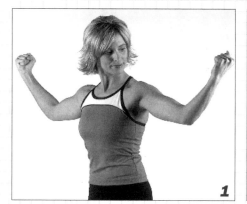 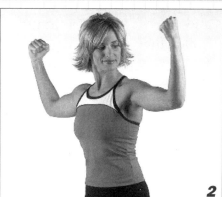 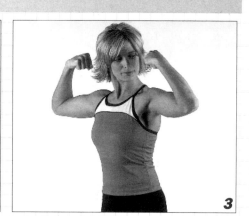

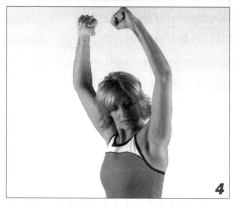 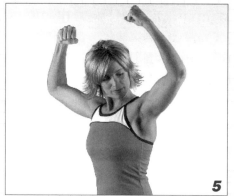 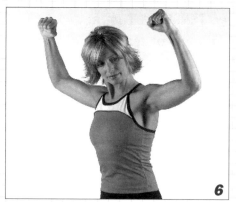

Stand with your feet at shoulder-width apart and arms extended (horizontally). From photo #1 move through photos #2-3, powerfully contracting biceps. Extend arms (vertically) with great tension as shown in photos #4-5. Return back to starting position under great tension (photo #6). Continue until you have completed 10 reps.

3. High Reach

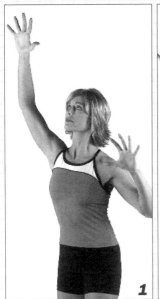
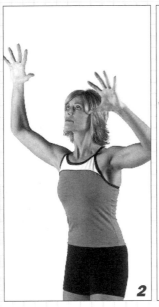
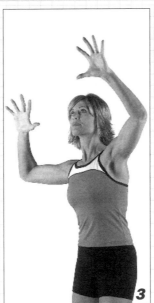
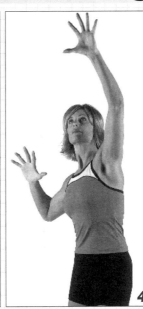

Stand with your feet at shoulder width and elbows bent, hands at shoulder height. Reach as high as possible while moving with great tension, one arm at a time. Use great tension in both directions. Palm can be open or hand can be clenched in tight fist to develop forearms.

4. One Arm Chin

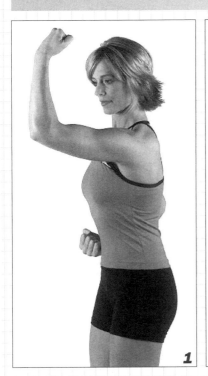
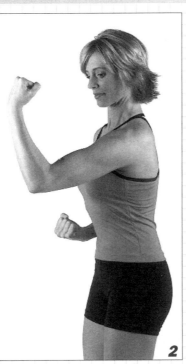
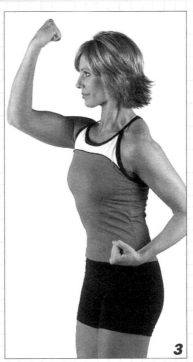

Stand with feet at shoulder width and hands in fists. Lift one arm above your head (see photo) and pull down with great tension (imagine doing a pull-up with one arm) toward the center-line of your body. As one arm pulls down move the other to the up position. Once again use great tension while pulling to the center line. 10 reps for each arm.

"It is not because things are difficult that we do not dare,
it is because we do not dare that they are difficult."

—Seneca

5. Full Range Pectoral Contraction

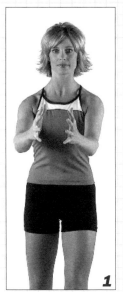 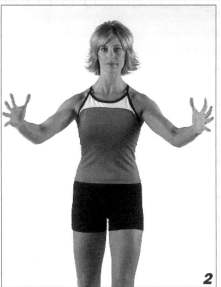 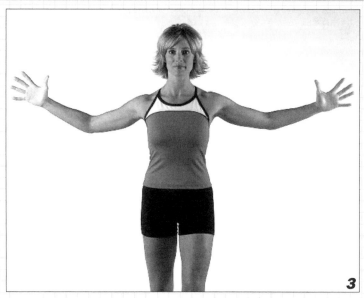

Stand with your left foot in front of your right foot and knee bent back straight (approximately one step, see photo). Hold hands in front, palms facing each other. Bring your hands back slowly with great tension until you feel your back muscles fully flexed. Hold for a count of one thousand one. Then move the hands slowly back to the original position while using great tension in your arms, shoulders, and pectoral muscles. Yes, the muscles will quiver.

6. Deltoid (Shoulder) Roll

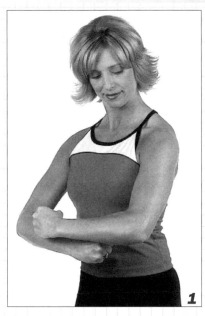 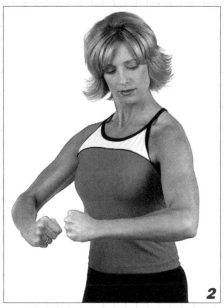 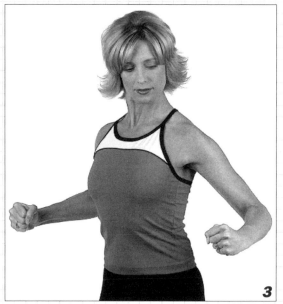

Stand with feet at shoulder width, knees slightly bent, and back straight. Hands in fists and both arms bent (see photo #1), roll arms and shoulders back until your back muscles are flexed. Hold for one thousand one. Then roll forward until your arms cross one on top of the other, right over left, then left over right, switching with each rep until you have completed 10 total reps (5 right over left, 5 left over right). Keep forearms parallel to the ground and shoulders low. This is a superb movement for the deltoids, arms, and pecs.

7. Wrist Twist Triceps Contraction

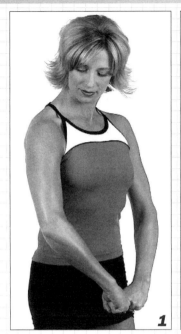
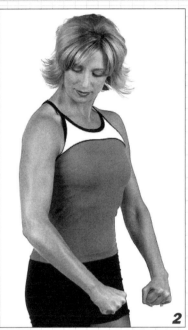
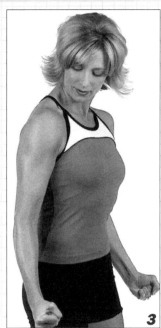

Stand with feet side-by-side, arms straight in front and close to your body (see photo #1), with fists turned in (backs of hands almost touching). Rotate arms as in photo #2, turning fists slowly until they turn out. Flex the back muscles and contract the triceps as hard as possible for one thousand one. Then slowly reverse arms, returning to the start position with great tension. Arms remain down and fully tensed during entire movement. 10 reps.

8. Deltoid Raise

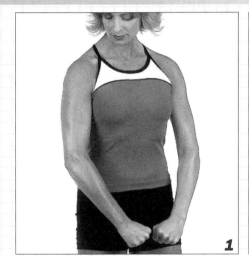
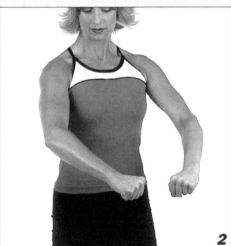

Feet side by side, hands in fists, feel tension in entire arm. Then slowly and with great tension raise your arms until they are extended overhead (photos #1-4). Reverse the movement, maintaining tension until your arms are at the starting position. *Don't just drop your arms!* Both movements should be done with great tension. 10 reps.

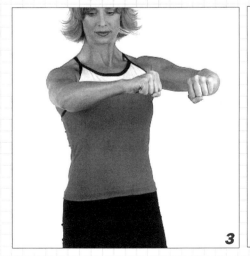
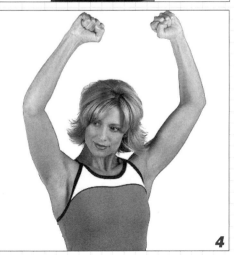

9. Biceps/Triceps Contraction

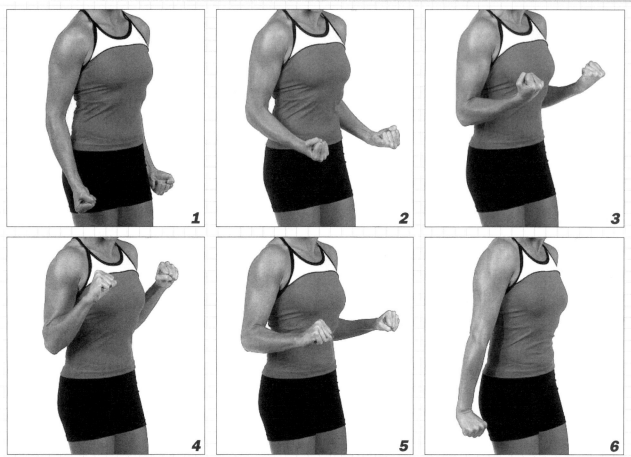

Standing with feet side by side, arms at sides, hands in tight fists facing forward (up), wrists flexed. Slowly and with great tension bend your elbows and curl your hands to your shoulders, contracting biceps as hard as possible. At top of movement reverse direction of your palms (palms point down, see photo #4) and slowly reverse direction and push down with great tension. At the bottom, flex your triceps hard. Reverse direction (palms up) and start the process once again. 10 reps.

10. Abdominal Contraction and Pull In (NOT PICTURED)

Stand with feet side by side, hands at sides. Press abdominal muscles down with great tension as you exhale. Flex muscles hard. Then pull in as hard as possible as you inhale forcefully. Create a strong vacuum. Hold for one thousand one. Continue for 10 reps, breathing with great force on both inhalation and exhalation.

11. Half Knee Bend

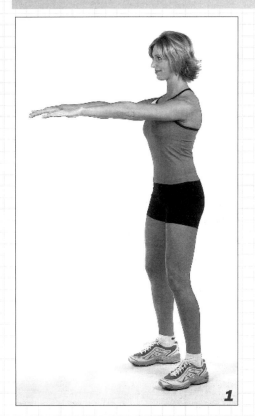 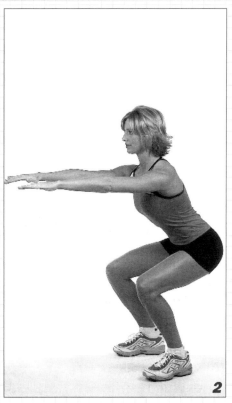 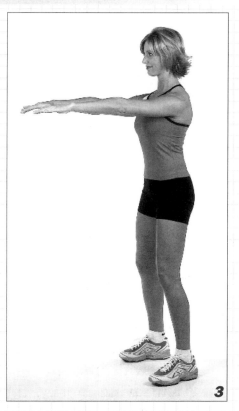

Stand with feet apart. Bend only halfway, but imagine you have a heavy weight across your shoulders. Feel extreme tension in the leg muscles as you slowly move down and up. Within a few weeks you will notice tremendous strength in your leg muscles and knee joints. 10 reps.

12. Calf Raise

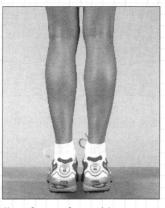 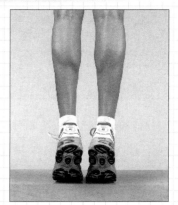

Stand with feet side by side. Have the balls of your feet either on a stair, a thick book, or even a piece of wood. Lower your heels and slowly raise up on your toes as high as possible with great tension. Lock your calves for just a moment at maximum tension, then slowly reverse direction and continue for 10 reps. Once you become adept at this exercise you can try doing it one leg at a time.

Question & Answer

Q: Do you really believe you can achieve as high a level of fitness at home as you can in a gym?

A: Absolutely! I used to go to a gym, and I've used a personal trainer, but I never achieved the definition, strength, and stamina—not to mention pain-free back—that I have with the *Transformetrics*™ program. I am saving money, time, and the results have been rewarding. Why do you need weights when God gave you all the equipment you need within your own body?

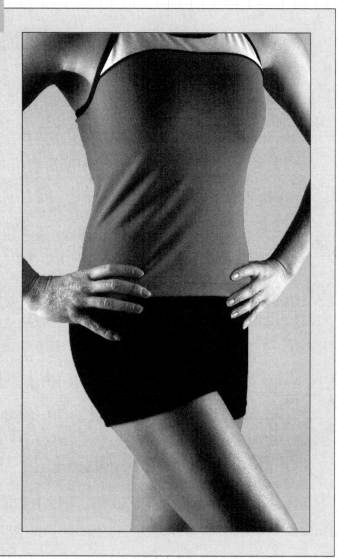

LESSON FOUR

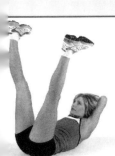
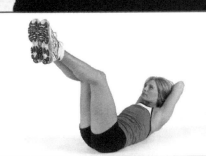
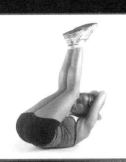

Abdominals

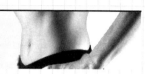

For some women, great abs are genetically inherited while others truly have to work hard to create and maintain ripped abs or even a flat tummy. I have several friends who never work on their abs and eat and drink what they want—they have no idea of how fortunate they are that genetics gave them this gift. For most women, including myself, this is an area we have to work hard at to achieve the results we want. It's not fair, but what are you going to do? It's sort of like the fact that some people are naturally better at certain subjects in school than others. You just have to work harder to succeed in your weak areas and enjoy the other areas that come more naturally. It's just the way life goes.

Abdominals are vital muscles to keep in shape as they are the core of your body and allow for a healthy posture and oppose the back muscles that are needed for the same purpose. To get the sculpted waistline that most women are trying to achieve, especially to get ready for the beach, you need to know which muscles make the difference: the rectus abdominis, external and internal obliques, and the overlooked TVA (transverse abdominis).

It seems as though everyone who is serious about fitness and exercise is interested in getting incredible abs. Keep in mind as you begin that the quality of the exercise is more important than the quantity for great looking abs. And remember that besides the obvious training of your abs, the other key is proper nutrition. You won't get the abs you want if you're playing fast and loose with your diet.

AB SCULPTING PROGRAM

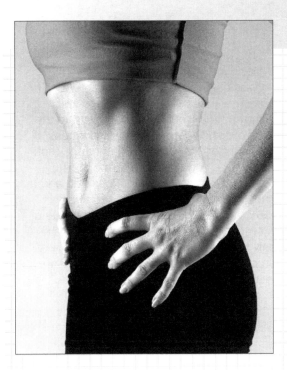

Are you ready for abs that scream, "I am in great shape!" Follow my ab exercises in this chapter and watch the heads turn. This program is second to none, and I found it to be sensitive to my lower back as well. I haven't had the back problems with these exercises I had in the past with other exercise systems. Remember to breathe out as you pull up and breathe in as you release. Breathing can make a huge difference in the development of the muscles. You will start to see results in no time flat.

The program is comprised of multiple variations of "The Crunch." The Crunch is a perfect example of exactly what I have already made reference to several times throughout this book. It is an exercise that combines Dynamic Self-Resistance and Dynamic Visualized Resistance. It can be made supremely difficult and effective by adding an Isometric Contraction at the very top of the movement or at the moment of strongest contraction. In fact, once you learn to "crunch" properly, it will help you master all forms of DSR and DVR.

THE POSITION

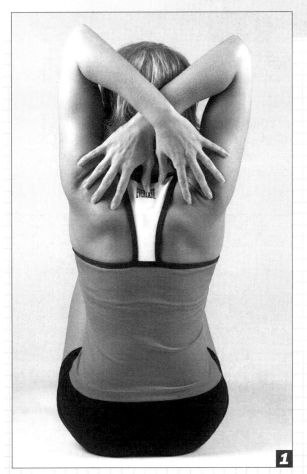

The *ideal position* for your hands in the performance of the Crunch is shown in photo #1. Please pay special attention to it.

If you are incapable of performing the exercise as in photo #1 due to neck pain or weakness, then use the following method that I devised for my friend Dr. Byron Armstrong. This method requires the use of a large bath towel. Study the photo #2 carefully. You will position yourself so that the towel extends below your buttocks and above your head. Then you will grab the two corners of the top of the towel as pictured. Your head and neck will be comfortably cradled, and you are now ready to begin.

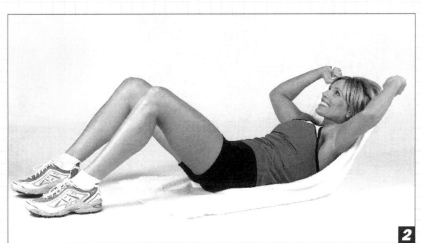

1

2

CR-1

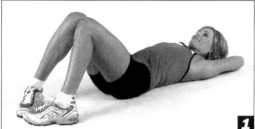
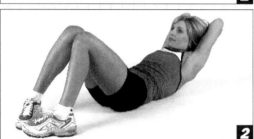

Lie on a carpeted floor or mat and place your hands either as shown in photo #1 or photo #2 from the previous page. Your knees will be bent with your feet about a foot from your hips. The knees are together, and feet should be positioned with toes as shown. With your lower back tight to the floor and pushing down, begin to roll your shoulders up. When your peak contraction is achieved, hold it for a count of "one thousand one, one thousand two." Then slowly and under complete control return to the starting position. This is one complete repetition. Start with 5 repetitions and add a maximum of one rep each week until you reach 10 reps per set. There is no need to ever go beyond 10 if you do these with deep concentration and with an isometric peak contraction on the last rep. This is also true in the 9 variations that follow, in which only the foot and leg positions vary. These changes emphasize different areas of the abdominal muscles and ensure you a complete workout for every aspect of the abdominal musculature.

CR-2

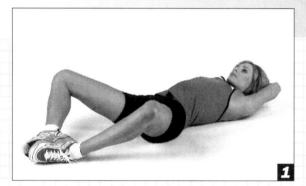
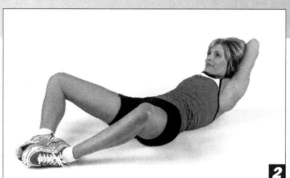

In this variation the lower abdominal and oblique muscles on the sides of the waist are affected by opening the knees wide and pressing the bottom of your feet together. As before, raise and lower, holding to peak contraction for a count of "one thousand one, one thousand two."

CR-3

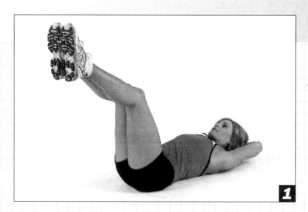
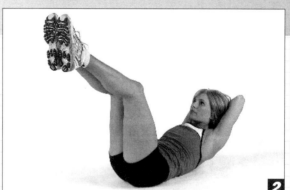

Raise your legs with your knees together and toes turned in to work the lower abdominal rows. Follow the same procedure as above, achieving peak contraction for a count of "one thousand one, one thousand two." Are you surprised by the intensity of 5 reps?

CR-4

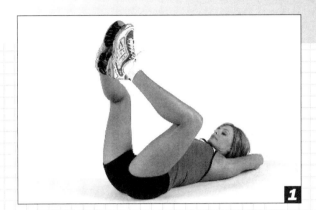 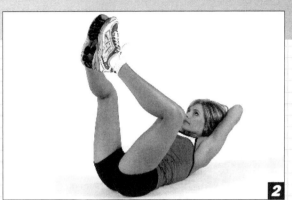

This variation exercises the obliques and lower abs from a new angle. Legs raised, knees opened wide, and place the bottom of your feet together. Once again, raise and hold your peak contraction, then lower.

CR-5

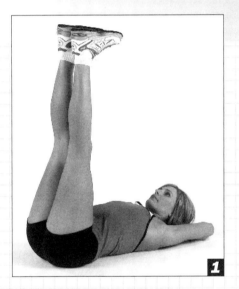 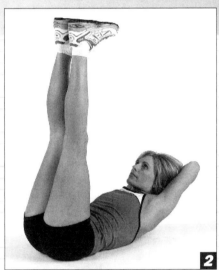

The center of the midsection is worked when the legs are straight up in the air. As in previous sets, slowly raise, contract deeply, and lower.

CR-6

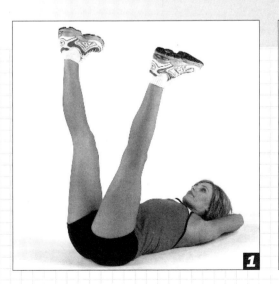 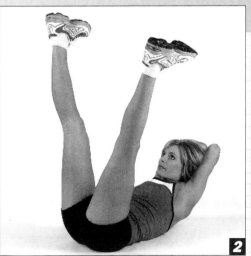

Lock the knees and spread the legs to work the upper abdominal row. Think about each repetition. Concentrate on the muscles being worked.

CR-7

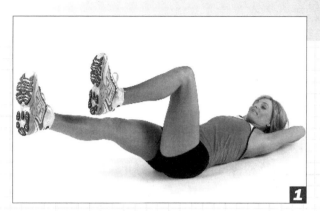
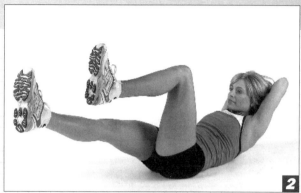

This is a very difficult variation, but the results are worth it. The left leg is held straight, six inches off the ground, while the right leg is bent 90 degrees. Switch position of legs and repeat.

CR-8

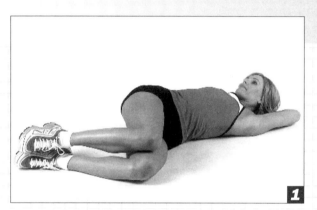
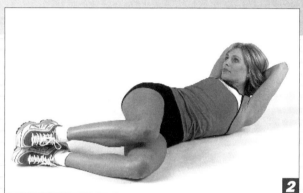

The obliques are worked by bending your knees and raising and lowering the upper body in a controlled turn at the waist. A partner may be used to help keep your knees down. Perform an equal number of repetitions on both sides of body.

CR-9

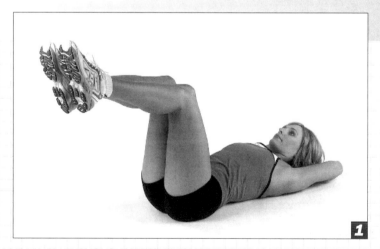
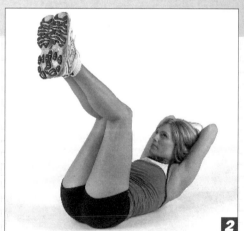

From position shown in photo #1, simultaneously raise shoulders and knees as shown in photo #2 holding peak contraction for "one thousand one, one thousand two."

CR-10

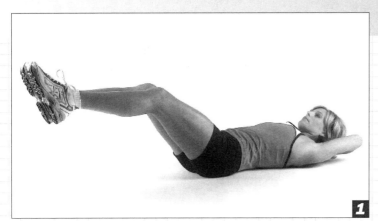 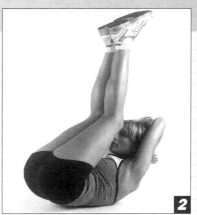

From position shown in photo #1, curl pelvis forward and raise and pull knees as close as possible to forehead, as shown in photo #2.

CR-11

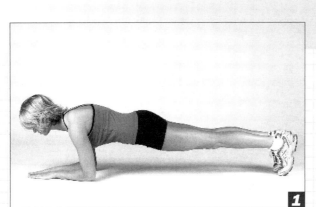 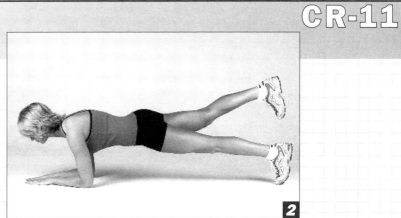

While holding your weight on your forearms and toes (in a plank position), lift your right leg off the floor about 12 to 18 inches while contracting abdominal muscles. Hold for 10 seconds. Repeat with left leg.

CR-12

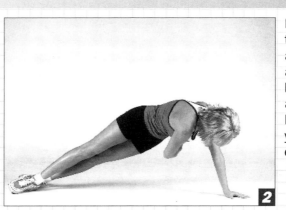

Hold a side plank position reaching your right arm to the ceiling. Rotate and twist your torso bringing your arm down and around your chest. Remember to hold in your abs. This is a great exercise for the obliques.

CR-13

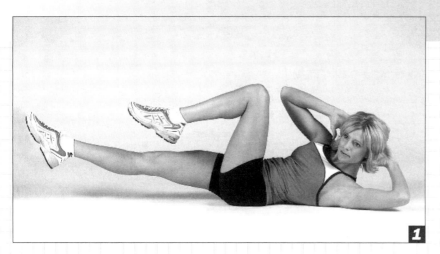

Start with one foot 6 inches off the floor while bringing one knee to the opposite elbow for a great oblique twist.

CR-14

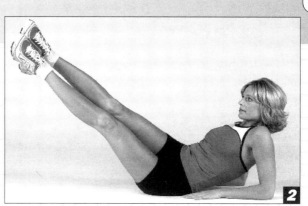

While on your back and up on your forearms, start with legs together, bent and twisted to the left. Then straighten your legs as shown in photo #2. Reverse on opposite side.

CR-15

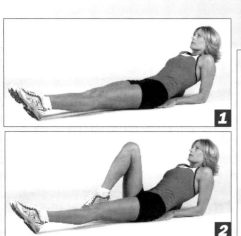

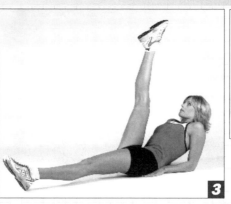

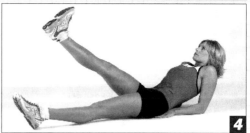

Start with legs straight on the floor, bringing right foot to left knee, preparing for extension. Keep abs tight throughout this exercise. Once extended, flex foot and use resistance to bring leg back to starting position. Reverse move with opposite leg.

CR-16

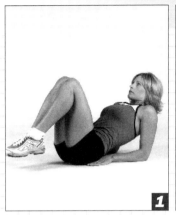 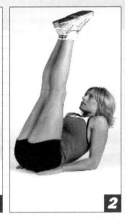 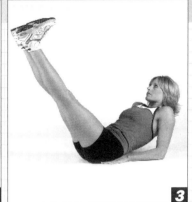 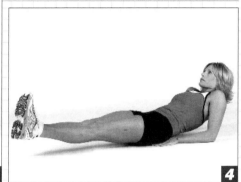

With legs together, bend at knees then extend in an upward motion. With flexed feet, resist on the downward movement finishing only 4 to 6 inches from the floor.

One More Thought...

"THE SILVER BULLET"

People ask me if there is a single ab exercise that does it all. Just one "silver bullet" that if practiced consistently would do the job. There is! And it's the exercise you see me performing here. It's called "The Superwoman Wheel Push-up." This one exercise truly does it all.

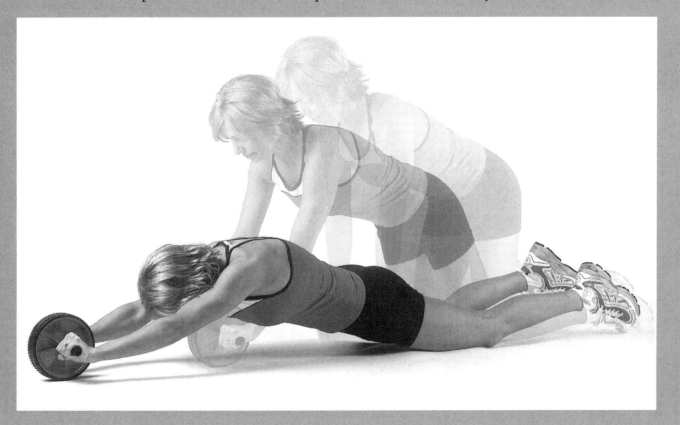

Question & Answer

Q: Will my muscles get used to this type of training and eventually "peak" at some point. I want to have the option of gaining mass or just keeping sculpted. Will *Transformetrics*™ allow for this flexibility?

A: With *Transformetrics*™ you will be able to achieve either a lithe, sculpted look, or you may gain mass if that is your desire. Since *Transformetrics*™ is based primarily on self-resistance, visualized resistance, and isometric training, there is really no room for "peaking." The goal is for you to achieve the look and size you desire, and then to maintain that. If you choose to add mass later, the same dynamics that got you to where you are come back into play. By adjusting the muscle tension you use as well as adjusting your diet, increased mass is always possible.

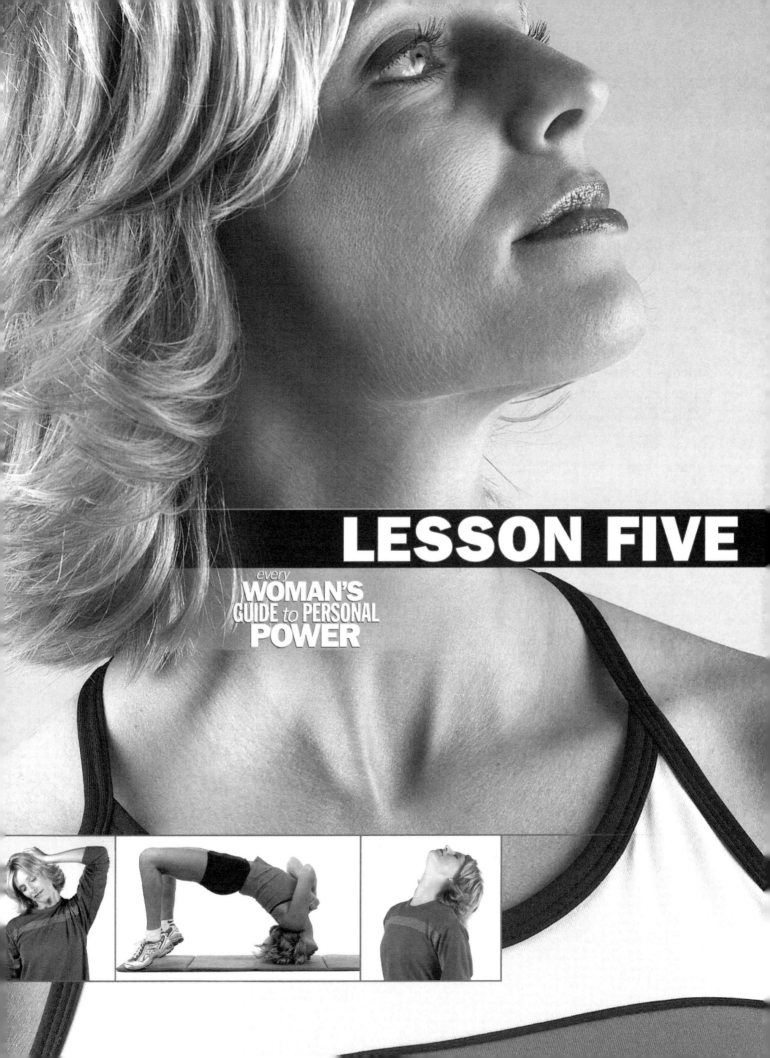

LESSON FIVE

every
WOMAN'S
GUIDE *to* **PERSONAL**
POWER

Neck

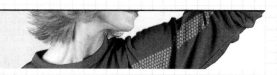

Women are obviously not interested in having the neck of an ox or the latest World Wrestling champion, but functional strength is another thing altogether. The neck is critically important in many sports and the neck muscles must be strong to gain the benefits your body can get from exercises such as the Furey Bridge. And let's face it, the neck helps to hold up the weight of our heads (approximately ten pounds, though sizes vary).

It's easy to forget that the first muscle group that everyone sees when they first meet us is our neck. A nicely developed neck can be a very attractive feature for a woman, especially if she has short hair or has long hair and pulls it up from time to time. If the neck is kept in shape, it will not show the early signs of aging as drastically as someone who never toned this particular body part. A turkey neck is definitely not appealing to the eye.

Be warned that you need to exercise the neck gradually and cautiously so that you don't end up with a sore, stiff neck. Very few people have developed the muscles of their neck properly.

NE-1 (DSR)
NECK FORWARD CONTRACTION

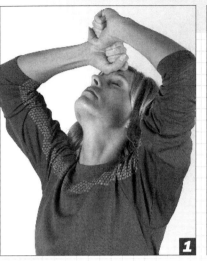 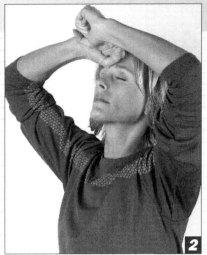

Bend your neck as far back as it will go and place your hands across your forehead. Now slowly bring your head forward and resist the movement slightly with your hands. Vary this by bringing your head slightly to the right and then slightly to the left, resisting with your hands. Repeat several times. As your strength increases, make the resistance more powerful. Once the neck muscles are acclimated, you may include isometric stops at various points in the range of motion. However, when you do so, gradually increase the resistance and gradually release resistance after 10 seconds.

NE-2 (DSR)
NECK BACKWARD CONTRACTION

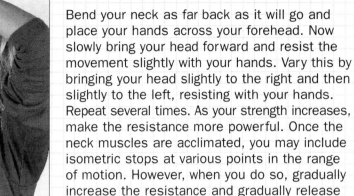

This exercise is the exact opposite of NE-1. The neck is bent forward with hands behind your head. Resist with your hands while endeavoring to force your head backward. When well conditioned, add isometric stops at any point you wish.

NE-3 (DSR)

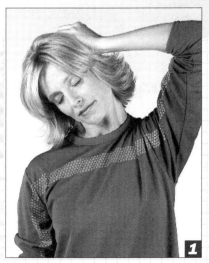 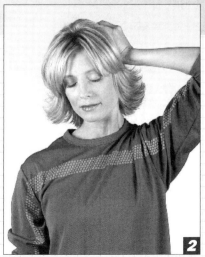

Bend your head to the right as close to the shoulder as is possible. Now place the left hand on the left side of your head and force your head to the left, resisting powerfully with the left hand. Try to touch your right ear to your left shoulder. Continue this 3 to 5 times. Then reverse the movement, beginning with the left ear to the left shoulder and moving your head to the right against the resistance of your right hand. Once again, after the muscles have become stronger, you may add 10-second isometric stops at any point in the range of motion.

NE-4 (DSR)

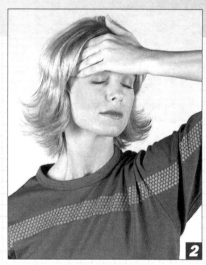

Turn your face to the left. Place your left hand on your forehead as pictured and resist while trying to turn your face to the right. Now turn your face to the right. Repeat 3 to 5 times. Now turn your face to the right and resist by placing your right hand on your forehead and endeavor to turn your face to the left against strong resistance. These are powerful exercises for the neck, and isometrics stops may be added.

NE-5 (DVR)

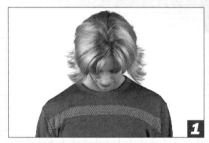
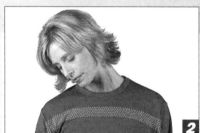
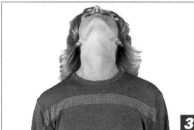
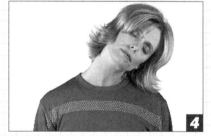

Anytime you do strength exercises for the neck, it is a good idea to end the session with neck rotation exercises to loosen and lubricate the neck joint. This is how it's done.

Bend your head far forward, chin on chest. Slowly bend around to the right, then backward and around to the left and around to the front. Make 3 to 5 complete rotations. Then reverse direction to the left. When doing this exercise, do it *slowly* and *vigorously* with tension. Don't do it so fast you get dizzy and end up falling down! That's a definite no.

NE-6 (DVR)

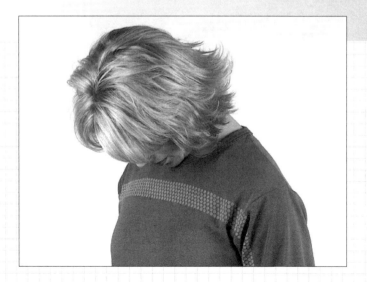

Throughout the day, the following exercise as well as NE-7 are excellent stress releasers. While standing, bend your head forward and carefully contract the front neck muscles as if trying to push your chin into your chest. Hold for a slow count of ten, then maintain your tension and slowly turn your face right as far as possible and then left. One complete rep is all that is necessary.

NE-7 (DVR)

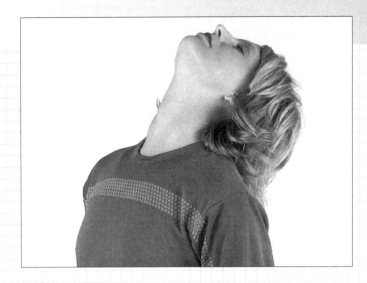

This is the same as NE-6 but in reverse. Bend your head far back and contract your neck muscles for a slow count of 10, then look right and left while maintaining the tension.

One More Thought...

The Furey Bridge is an amazing exercise in that it uses a combination of power calisthenics and isometric contractions. You'll love the flexibility you gain from doing this exercise. With this particular isometric your goal should be to hold this position for 3 minutes or longer. I personally also find this exercise to be an excellent tool for meditating.

Notice the wrong way that has been pictured. Work your way to getting your forehead and nose to the mat. You will be amazed at its effectiveness.

NE-8 (PC/ISO)
THE FUREY BRIDGE

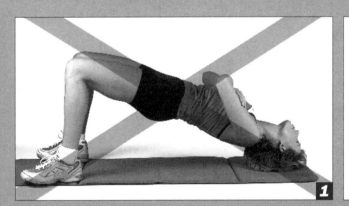

Photo 1 shows the **wrong way**.

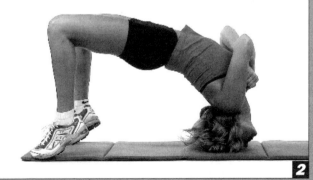

Photo 2 shows the **Furey way**. I know it seems extreme, but once you work up to it, your flexibility will be nothing less than incredible and wall walking will seem like child's play—because, by comparison, it is!

Question & Answer

Q: I am 68 and have tried several workout systems in the past. Some work and some do not. I am a little flabby, thanks to my age and lack of exercise in recent months. Am I too old to start *Transformetrics*™, and will I see the flab disappear?

A: It's never too early or too late in life to start *Transformetrics*™. This program will actually help you maintain muscles that you already have or increase what does not exist as well as lose the flab. *Transformetrics*™ will help slow down bone loss and help keep your heart healthy. If you have any form of arthritis, this program will also help, because it does not put any stress on the joints.

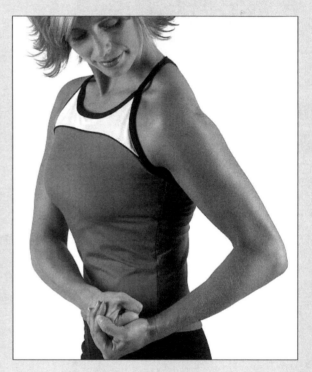

LESSON SIX

every
WOMAN'S
GUIDE *to* **PERSONAL**
POWER

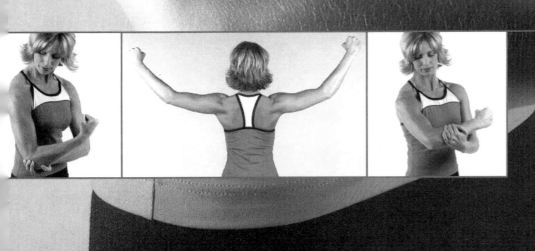

Shoulders

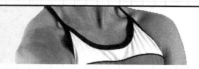

O ne of the big "pluses" of the *Transformetrics*™ program for me personally has been to have friends say, "Wow, Wendie! What have you been doing to get your shoulders to look like that?" Up until the first person said that to me, it hadn't dawned on me the difference *Transformetrics*™ made in the muscular definition of my shoulders. But it did! And I couldn't help but smile when I looked in the mirror and saw it for myself. I had never been complimented on my shoulders before that. Now it's almost a daily occurrence.

I can tell you from my shoulder injury that you need to pay special attention to the development of your shoulder muscles. There are seventeen muscles working in your shoulders, and you can't afford for any of them to be weak. These exercises will do the trick and develop them all.

What I am about to show you in this chapter will allow you to develop "sexy," strong shoulders for sundress season, tennis, golf, or anytime you may find yourself going sleeveless. These exercises build, strengthen, and help with flexibility as well as rounding out the muscles of your shoulders. So, if you're ready, let's go and beautify your shoulders!

SH-1 (DVR)
McSWEENEY HIGH REACH

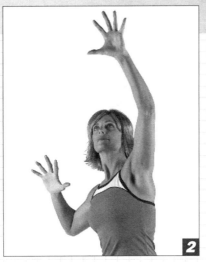

Stand with your feet shoulder-width apart and elbows bent, hands at shoulder height. One arm at a time, reach as high as possible while moving against great tension. Maintain maximum tension in both directions. Palm can be open or hand can be clenched in a tight fist to develop your forearms.

SH-1A (DVR)
HIGH REACH W/ LUNGE

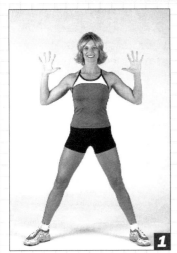 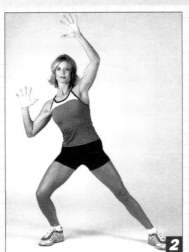 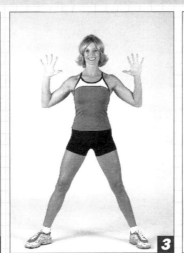 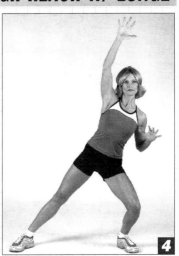

SH-2 (DVR)
SHOULDER ROLL

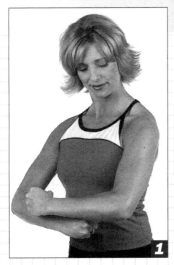 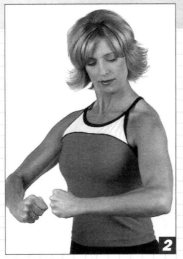

Stand with your feet at shoulder width, knees bent slightly, back straight, hands in fists, and one hand over the other as pictured (arms bent). From this position, roll your arms and shoulders back until your back muscles are fully flexed. Your arms should remain bent throughout the range of motion. Hold for "one thousand one," maintaining maximum tension. Then roll forward until your arms cross one on top of the other, right over left and then left over right, switching with each repetition until you have completed 10 repetitions (5 right over left, 5 left over right). Keep your forearms parallel to the ground and shoulders low. This is a superb movement for the deltoids, arms, and pecs.

SH-3 (DVR)
DELTOID RAISE

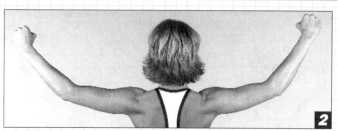

Stand with your feet side by side, arms at front, fists clenched, wrists flexed. Against maximum tension, *slowly* raise your arms outward and upward until they reach the position shown (do not fling them). At this point think into and powerfully contract your deltoid (shoulder) muscles. This is great for stretching and limbering up. Do it often.

SH-4 (DSR)
FRONT DELTOID CONTRACTION

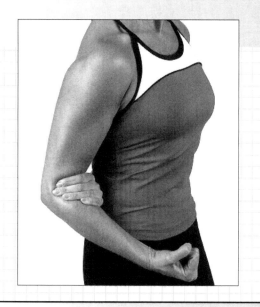

Allow your right arm to hang at your side and slightly backward. Now grasp the inside elbow (see photo) from the back by your left hand and endeavor to pull your right arm far forward, resisting powerfully with the left hand. This is a very short movement, only a few inches, but nonetheless a very powerful and result-producing exercise. Switch sides and continue.

SH-5 (DSR)

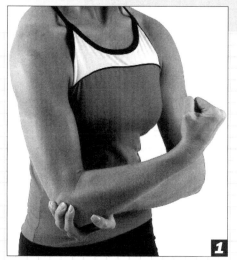
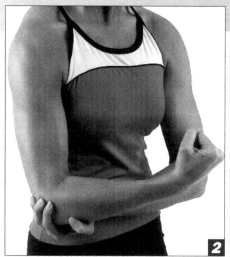

Bring your right elbow across the chest and grasp your elbow firmly with your left hand. Slowly force the right arm downward and backward against the powerful resistance supplied by your left hand. Repeat until fatigued, then switch arms and continue. This exercise strengthens the back of the shoulders.

SH-6 (DSR)

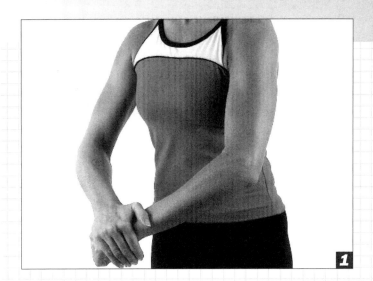

Grasp your left hand with the right hand in front (see photo). Gradually raise your entire arm outward and upward against the powerful resistance of your right hand. Repeat until fatigued, then switch arms and continue. Superb for outer shoulder muscles.

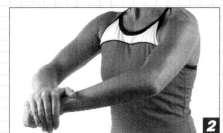

SH-7 (DSR)

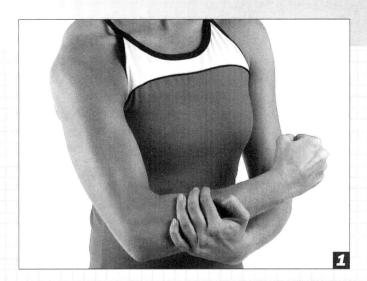

Bend your right arm as pictured. Now grasp your right forearm from underneath and raise your arm outward and upward against the resistance of your left arm. This is a powerful movement for side deltoids.

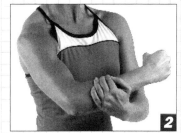 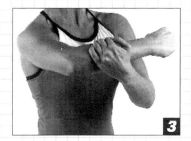

SH-8 (DSR)

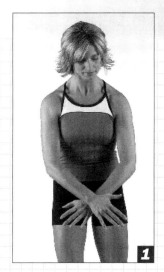 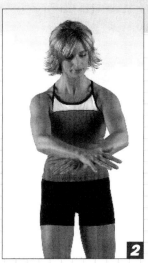 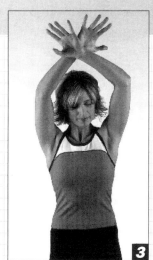

With your arms straight, place your right hand over your left hand as pictured. Against the resistance of your right hand pulling down, raise your left arm until both arms are straight overhead. Reverse directions and lower against resistance. Switch to your left hand on top of the right and continue. With enough resistance, 3 to 5 reps is plenty.

SH-9 (DSR)

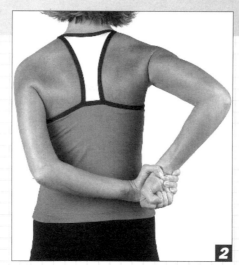

Place your right arm down against your side with your hand slightly behind the centerline of your body. Grasp your right wrist with your left hand in back of you. Raise your right shoulder as high and as slowly as possible while resistance is powerfully applied by your left hand pulling downward. Switch sides when fatigued and continue. Remember, you must use strength to build strength. This powerful exercise is for the trapezius at the top of the shoulder.

SH-10 (ISO)

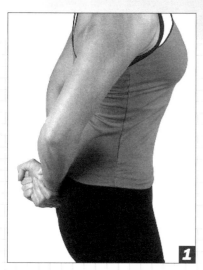 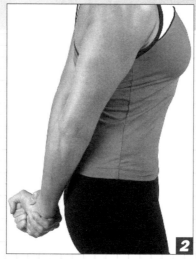

While standing with your arms behind your back, grasp your right wrist with your left hand. Slowly endeavor to straighten your right hand out and down. Now, while building tension to the limit, breathe in deeply, and then at the peak of the contraction slowly exhale making an "ssss" sound, counting to 10. Gradually ease tension. Repeat, grasping your left wrist with your right hand.

Only one maximum tension isometric is necessary from both sides. But remember— slowly build the tension and hold at the maximum, then slowly release.

SH-11 (ISO)
SAMSON PRESS OUT

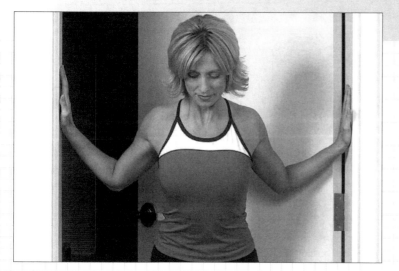

Your hands should be flat against the sides of the doorjamb at shoulder height. Press out while breathing in and build to maximum tension. Once at maximum tension, breathe out slowly ("ssss" sound) while maintaining for 10 seconds. Relax your tension slowly.

SH-12 (ISO)
LATERAL RAISE

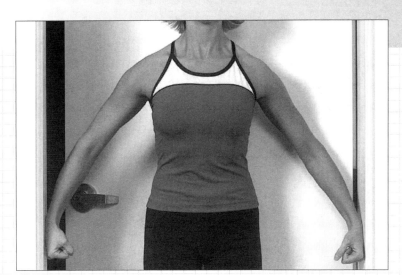

Do this one exactly as pictured. Build your tension to a maximum while breathing in. Hold your tension while slowly exhaling to a slow count of 10. Then slowly ease off the tension.

SH-13 (ISO)
BRINGIN' DOWN THE HOUSE

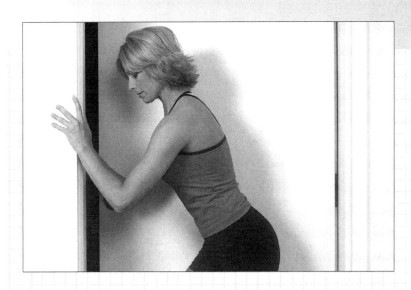

Position yourself as shown in the photo. Slowly build to maximum tension while breathing in. Hold your tension at the peak contraction while slowly breathing out.

Question & Answer

Q: I try to eat right every day, but on hectic days it's almost impossible to get in a nutritious lunch. Do you have any suggestions?

A: Despite our busyness, we have to make the most of what goes into our bodies even in crunch time. If you can't get in a nutritious meal, I suggest you take a Revival Soy protein drink as a nutritious substitute. Try their low carb bars, too. It would be better to do this than to deprive your body of food altogether. On page 55 there is more information on Revival products as well as an ordering code to make it easy. Soy actually curbs your appetite while supplying you with the nutrients your body needs.

One More Thought...

I want to encourage you that even if you do no other power calisthenics, do as many Furey Push-ups as possible every day. It is the single best exercise known for creating strength, flexibility, and endurance in the entire shoulder muscle structure.

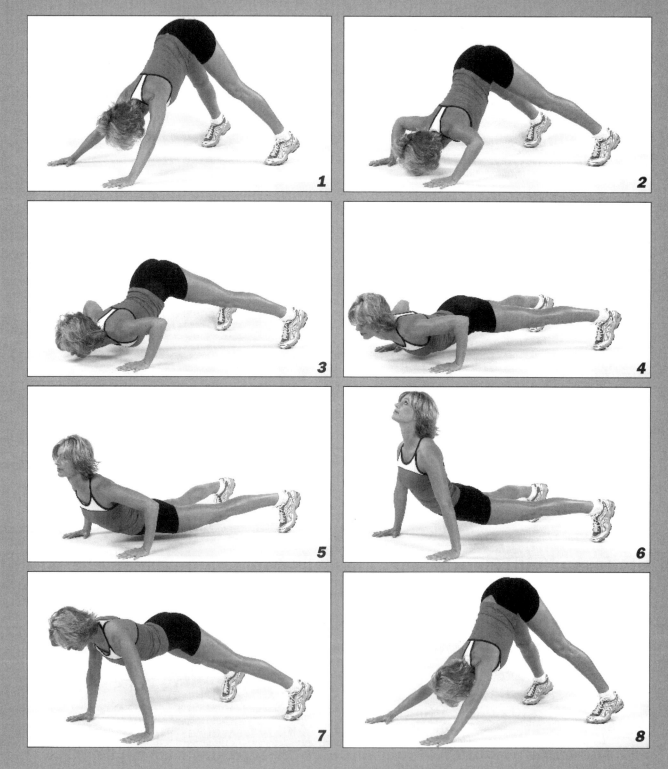

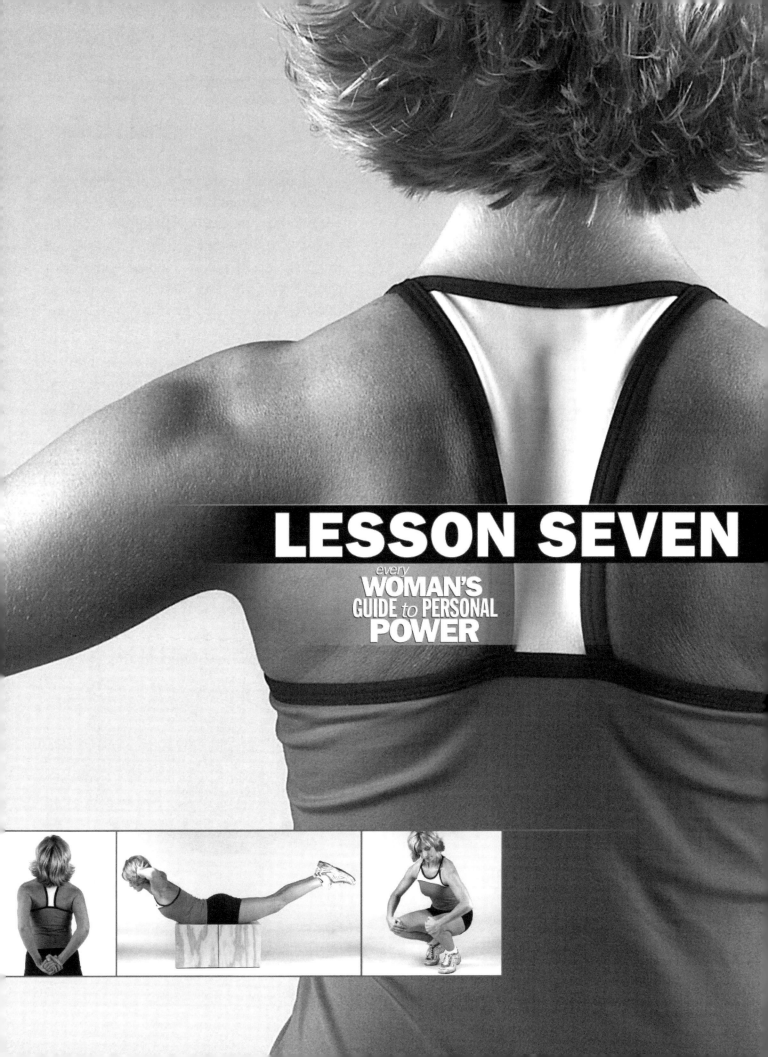

LESSON SEVEN

every
WOMAN'S
GUIDE *to* **PERSONAL**
POWER

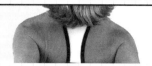

Back

A strong supple back is something every woman aspires to, but most of us don't have a clue when it comes to knowing how to achieve it. In looking back, I can see that I didn't even realize how weak my back was and how it was contributing to my back pains. Prior to turning to *Transformetrics™*, I could have never done a single pull-up or chin-up without assistance. Now I can do several, and I'm amazed!

A member on the Bronze Bow Publishing web site forum named Duff, a lean gentleman who stands 6'5", stated that before he started *Transformetrics™* his maximum for pull-ups was five in a row. Since he started *Transformetrics™*, which had only been three months, he could do ten pull-ups in a row without assistance and hardly a struggle. That is a 100 percent increase in only three months, which speaks volume. On top of this accomplishment, he added ten pounds of pure muscle to his physique in the same three months.

It is very possible that you have tried different forms of training that not only left you drained but also in an injured state. Having strong healthy back muscles helps prevent osteoporosis and prepares the back for the pressure of childbearing. Without a strong back you will typically suffer from sleepless nights and achy days.

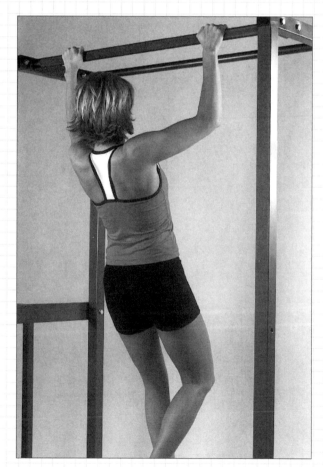

BA-1 (DSR)

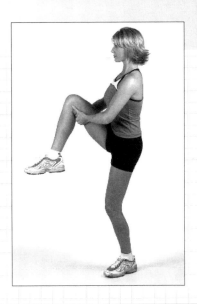

Grasp both hands around your right thigh, as shown, just above the knee. Then with both arms pulling up, resist powerfully with the thigh. Perform 3 to 5 repetitions with extreme tension, then switch to your left thigh and do 3 to 5 more. This exercise is a powerful conditioner of both the upper and lower back muscles.

BA-2 (DSR)

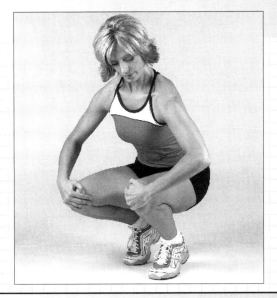

While in a squat position (see photo), place your hands on the inside of your knees and then pull the knees apart while resisting powerfully with the legs pulling in. This movement is superb for the upper back, shoulders, and arms and also makes the muscles of the inner thigh more shapely. 3 to 5 ultra-tension repetitions are all that is required.

BA-3 (DVR/ISO)

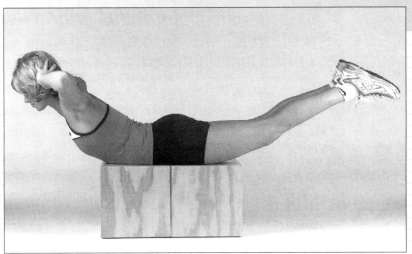

While lying face down across a cushioned stool or chair, hands clasped behind your neck, simultaneously bend your head and feet upward. This is a very short movement. When your peak contraction is reached on your third to fifth repetition, try to hold for a 10-second isometric. At this point think into and powerfully contract your deltoid (shoulder) muscles. This is great for stretching and limbering up. Do it often.

BA-4 (DVR)

Same position as BA-3 but with your hands now placed at lower back. First, bend the left side of your upper body upward (hold contraction for "one thousand one"), return to starting position, and then raise your body to the right. Repeat 3 to 5 times on each side. This will be difficult at first, but you'll be pleased with the results.

BA-5

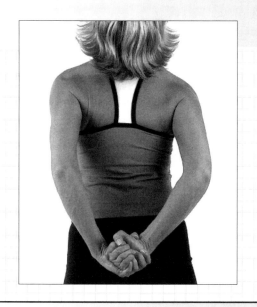

Grasp your hands behind your back. Push your shoulders downward and backward and bend your head and back as far back as you can while powerfully tensing all of the muscles of both your back and neck. Hold peak contraction for a slow count of 10. 3 to 5 repetitions.

BA-6 (DVR)
FUREY WALL WALK

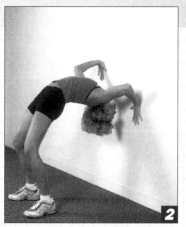
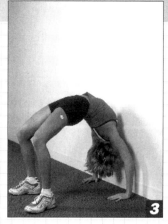

Stand 18" to 24" from a wall with your arms fully extended above your head. Slowly bend backward under complete control, touch the wall, and then walk hands downward until touching the floor with your palms. Perform slowly and feel your muscles contract and then stretch.

BA-7 (DVR)

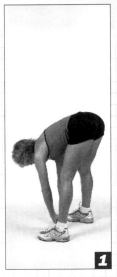 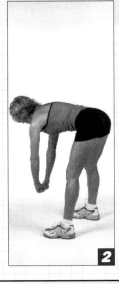 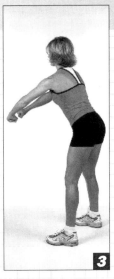 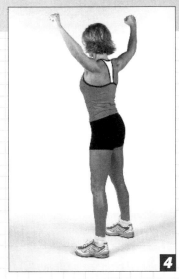

With feet about 20" apart, bend down and touch the floor. As you come back up, fling your arms outward, upward, and backward as far as they will go. Repeat frequently throughout the day.

BA-8 (ISO)

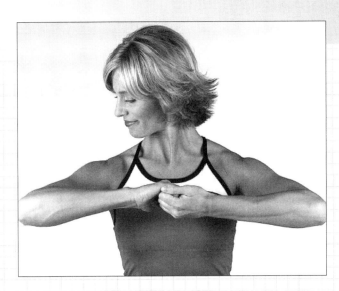

With your hands directly in front of your chest, clasp your hands as shown—your left hand facing your chest (thumb and forefinger in up position), your right hand facing out (thumb and forefinger down). While breathing in, slowly build pressure as you pull outward to the maximum. At the peak contraction, slowly breathe out making an "ssss" sound. Hold the contraction for 10 seconds and slowly release. Breathe deeply. When recovered, reverse hand positions and repeat. Only 1 repetition of each hand position is required.

BA-9 (ISO)

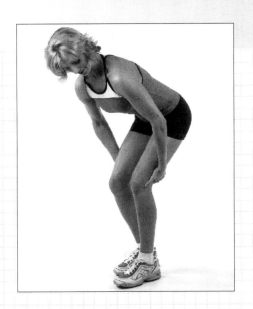

While standing, lean forward and wrap your arms around your legs just above the knees, clasping your hands together. Attempt to lift your legs with your arms. Endeavor to lift from the shoulders and upper back to avoid placing undue stress on the lower back.

BA-10 (ISO)

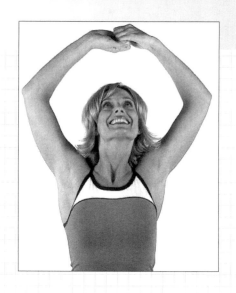

With your arms straight above your head (as shown) and as far back as possible, grip your hands (left palm down, right palm up). Attempt to pull your hands apart. Follow standard isometric procedure. After completion, reverse grip and do one more repetition.

BA-11 (ISO)

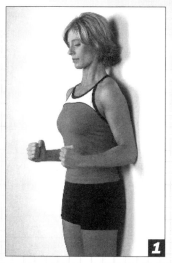 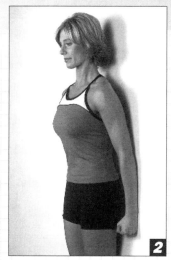

Stand with your back against a wall, arms bent as shown in photo #1. Push the back of your arms against the wall and hold peak contraction 10 seconds.

Photo #2—Repeat with arms in position shown.

BA-12 (ISO)

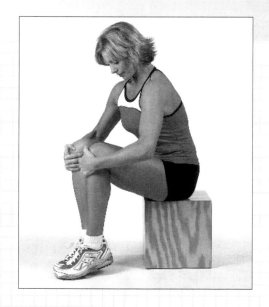

While seated, raise up on your toes as shown and place your hands around the fronts of your knees. With your fingers pointed inward and curling around your knees, pull straight back as forcefully as possible while simultaneously trying to lower your heels to the floor. Hold peak isometric contraction for 10 seconds. This one is great for the lats, abs, and forearms.

BA-13 (ISO)

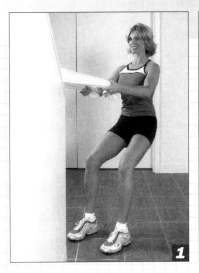 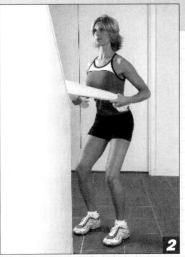

Loop a towel around a stationary object. Pull out and down while in a half-squat position, slowly pull yourself forward contracting through the pull. Hold this position for 10 seconds. Gradually ease the tension.

One More Thought...

In the beginning, resistence bands may be a useful tool until you get the feel of "thinking into your muscles," without the bands. You may use bands of this type on numerous exercises throughout this book.

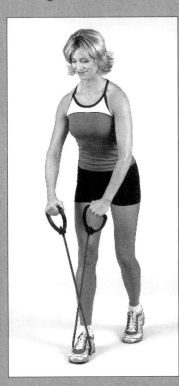 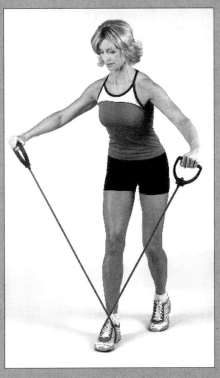 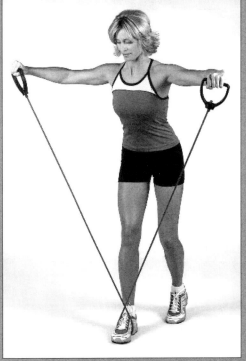

One More Thought...

I was honestly never able to perform chin-ups or pull-ups until I practiced the *Transformetrics*™ program. (That was prior to being injured) Now, only one year later from a shoulder injury I can do these exercises in amazement. *You can too!*

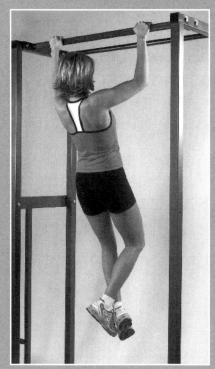

Wide Grip Pull-Up

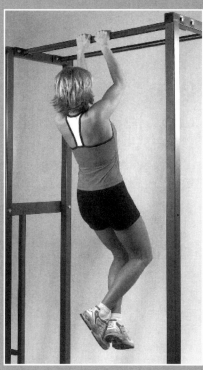

Close Grip Pull-Up

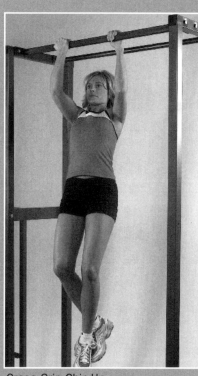

Cross Grip Chin-Up

LESSON EIGHT

every
WOMAN'S
GUIDE *to* **PERSONAL**
POWER

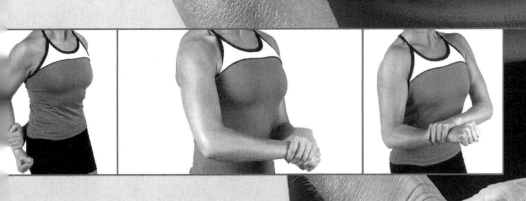

Biceps

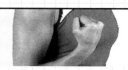

Having lean, muscular arms seems to be a common goal for women. However, unless you are genetically gifted, developing nicely toned biceps takes time and effort. Consistent *Transformetrics*™ training, cardiovascular exercise, proper nutrition, and adequate rest are all essential for shapely biceps.

Your biceps muscles will vary in shape due to your genetic makeup and the distance from your shoulder to your elbow. For instance, I have really long arms for my height, so my muscles aren't built into the "ball look" as someone may get if they have shorter arms with little distance between their shoulder and elbow.

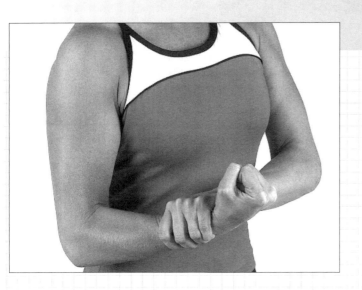

BI-1 (DSR)
BICEPS CURL

Grasp your right wrist with your left hand. Your right hand is in a tight fist, palm up. You want to flex your wrist to engage the forearm muscles. Against the powerful resistance from your left arm, slowly curl your right fist to your right shoulder. Switch to your left side and continue.

REPETITIONS	
MODERATE	10
HEAVY	6-8
VERY HEAVY	3-5

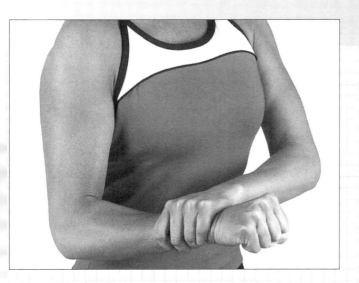

BI-2 (DSR)
REVERSE BICEPS CURL

Same as above except that your fist is in a palm-down position.

REPETITIONS	
MODERATE	10
HEAVY	6-8
VERY HEAVY	3-5

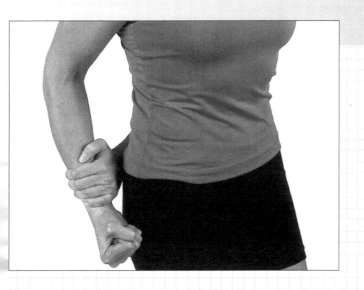

BI-3 (DSR)
CURL FROM BEHIND

With your right arm down at your side and slightly to the rear, place your left hand in your right palm from behind and curl your right hand toward your right shoulder against the powerful resistance supplied by your left arm. This is a very powerful movement. Switch sides and continue.

REPETITIONS	
MODERATE	10
HEAVY	6-8
VERY HEAVY	3-5

BI-4 (DSR)

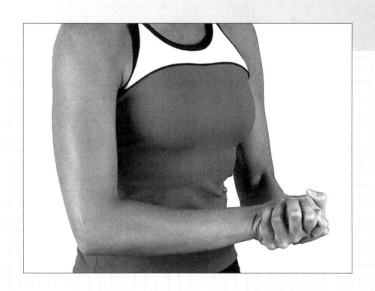

Grasp your hands in front, your left palm up and right palm down. Against powerful resistance, curl your left arm to your left shoulder. On the downward motion, resist strongly with your left hand, thus exercising the right triceps muscle. Study the photos and note that both arms have excellent leverage in this position. Switch arms and continue right palm up, left palm down.

REPETITIONS	
MODERATE	10
HEAVY	6-8
VERY HEAVY	3-5

BI-5 (DSR)

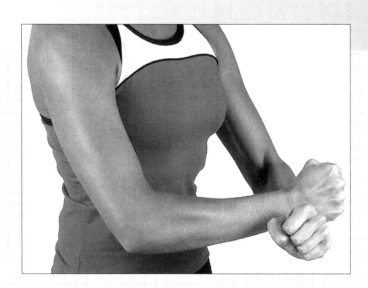

Same as BI-4 except your hands are clenched in fists, one over the other (see photo). Superb leverage allows you to apply maximum resistance from both arms. Switch arm position to left over right and continue.

REPETITIONS	
MODERATE	10
HEAVY	6-8
VERY HEAVY	3-5

BI-6 (DSR)

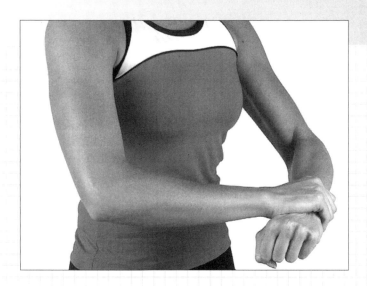

Same position as BI-4 only with palms down. Use powerful resistance. Switch arm positions and continue.

REPETITIONS	
MODERATE	10
HEAVY	6-8
VERY HEAVY	3-5

BI-7 (DSR)

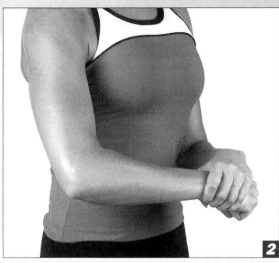

With your right upper arm at your side and your forearm across your chest, place your left hand over the back of your right wrist. Against powerful resistance, slowly raise your right forearm outward and upward. Your upper arm remains as close to your side as possible and does not rise at the shoulder. This is superb for the side muscle of the upper arm. Switch arms and continue.

BI-8 (DVR)

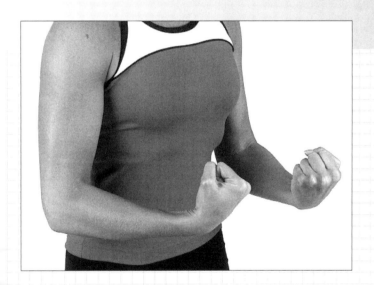

Clench your fists tightly and slowly curl both arms to your shoulder against visualized resistance, contracting your biceps as tightly as possible at the top of the movement. On the downward movement, turn the palms of your fist down and slowly extend. At the bottom of the movement, contract your triceps as strongly as possible. Continue on.

REPETITIONS	
MODERATE	10
HEAVY	6-8
VERY HEAVY	3-5

BI-9 (DVR)
CONCENTRATION CURL

While seated as pictured with your elbow on your right thigh, slowly curl your right fist to your right shoulder. Contract the biceps powerfully at the top of the movement. Continue and then switch arms.

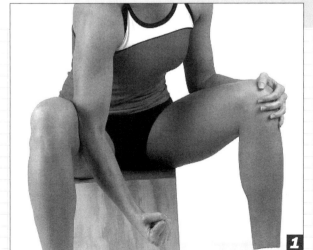

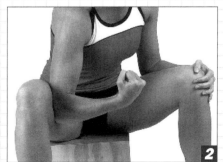

REPETITIONS	
MODERATE	10
HEAVY	6-8
VERY HEAVY	3-5

BI-10 (DVR)
ATLAS BICEPS FLEX AND PRESS

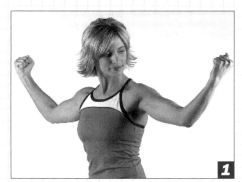
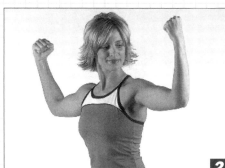
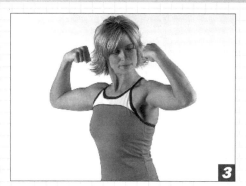
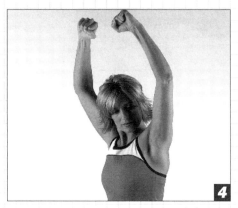
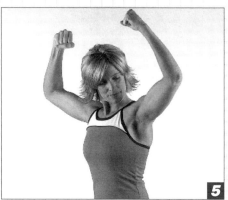
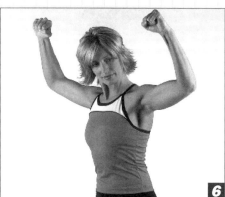

Stand with your feet at shoulder-width apart and arms extended (horizontally). From photo #1 move through photos #2-3, powerfully contracting biceps. Extend arms (vertically) with great tension as shown in photos #4-5. Return back to starting position under great tension (photo #6). Continue until you have completed 10 reps.

BI-11 (DVR)
(NOT PICTURED)

With your right fist close to your right shoulder, practice powerfully contracting and then relaxing the biceps. This is a short but powerful movement. Repeat with your left arm.

One More Thought...

In addition to the biceps exercises found here, keep in mind that all forms of chin-ups and pull-ups work the biceps and forearms powerfully. If you currently have difficulty doing pull-ups, you won't after doing these exercises for a few months.

LESSON NINE

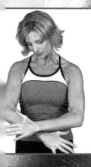
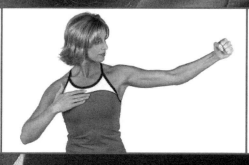
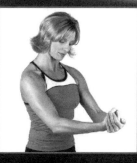

Triceps

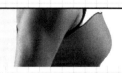

*I*n general, women have stronger biceps than triceps muscles. The triceps muscle has a horseshoe appearance on the back of the upper arm. You need to develop both biceps and triceps in conjunction with one another for a more appealing healthy look. Triceps are typically easy to develop, but most women are only aware of a couple of exercises to perform. In this chapter I will show you over ten *Transformetrics*™ moves to practice for the triceps. Remember, all of the push-ups and pull-ups require triceps concentration as well.

TR-1 (DSR)
BLADE HAND PRESS OUT

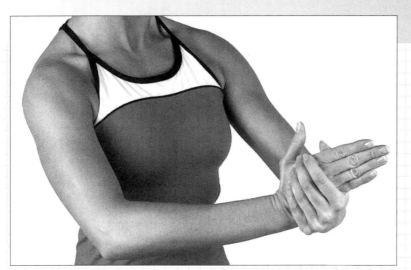

With your right hand held as shown in the photo and with great power, slowly extend your right arm from just under your chin (elbows down) to a complete extension. Your left biceps is powerfully exercised during the resistance phase. A maximum of 3 to 5 reps is all that is required. Switch and repeat with your left hand. The superb leverage of this exercise makes it excellent.

REPETITIONS	
MODERATE	10
HEAVY	6-8
VERY HEAVY	3-5

TR-2 (DVR)
McSWEENEY WRIST TWIST

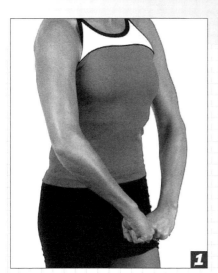

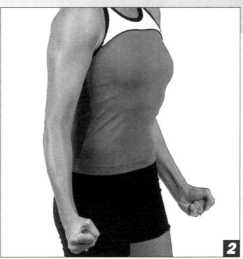

With arms in front as shown and backs of hands almost touching, slowly and with great tension rotate your arms back, turning the fists gradually until they turn out completely. At this point the triceps and upper back muscles are flexed powerfully, and you need to try to flex even harder for a count of "one thousand one," then slowly return to the starting position with great tension. If you exert extreme tension, 3 to 5 reps is all that is necessary.

TR-3 (DSR)
TRICEPS EXTENSION

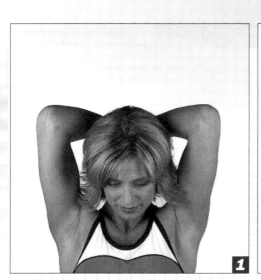

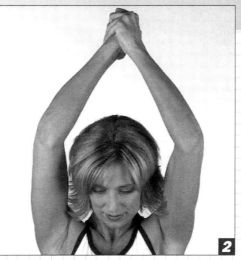

Using the same grip as TR-1 except that your elbows are bent and both hands start behind your neck (see photo), press up and outward against extreme tension for 3 to 5 reps. Switch hands and repeat.

REPETITIONS	
MODERATE	10
HEAVY	6-8
VERY HEAVY	3-5

TR-4 (DVR)
THE C.A.T. (CHEST, ABS, TRICEPS)

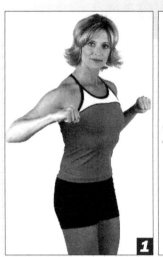 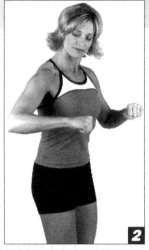 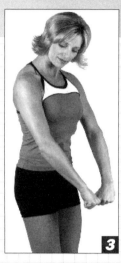

Stand straight with your feet at shoulder-width apart. Start by bringing both hands (fists palm down) to shoulder level with your elbows lower. Push down with great tension. This is done by consciously contracting the biceps while extending down with your triceps. Extend down below waist level and slightly bend your knees. This exercise is superb for the pectorals, abs, biceps, and especially triceps. If you practice in front of a mirror, you will see that you are exercising your muscles in unison.

TR-5 (DSR)
BACK FIST DOWN

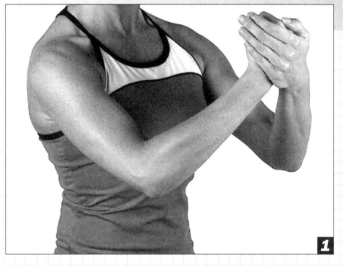

Hold your right fist palm up in your left hand. Slowly extend your right arm out and down against the strong resistance of your left hand pulling up and toward you. Switch and repeat, extending your left back fist and pulling with your right hand.

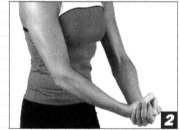

REPETITIONS	
MODERATE	10
HEAVY	6-8
VERY HEAVY	3-5

TR-6 (DVR)
CROSSING HANDS

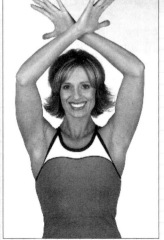 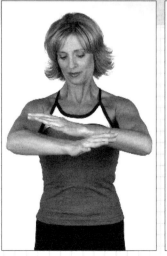 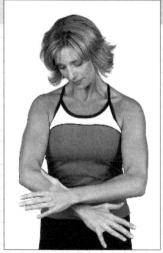

Take a good look at the photos. This exercise is done at 3 levels, and each repetition the relative position of the hands changes—left over right, right over the left, 3 to 5 reps in each of the 3 positions. This is a powerful exercise for the abs, chest, biceps, and triceps, which receive an especially concentrated workout.

REPETITIONS	
MODERATE	10
HEAVY	6-8
VERY HEAVY	3-5

TR-7 (DSR)
TRICEP PUSH DOWN

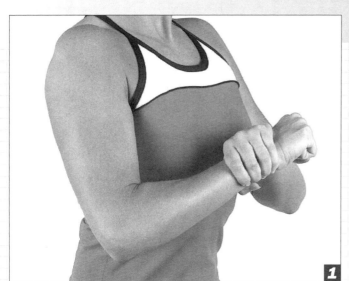

Hold arms as shown (upper arms remain close to body throughout movement), left hand clasping back of right fist at centerline of body. While resisting powerfully with right arm, push down and out with left hand. After completing one set, reverse arms right over left. This is a very powerful exercise—don't neglect it.

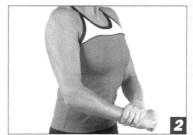

REPETITIONS	
MODERATE	10
HEAVY	6-8
VERY HEAVY	3-5

TR-8 (DVR)
VERTICAL PALM PRESS

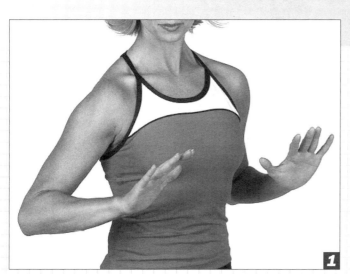

With your hands at chest level and palms forward (see photo #1), push out slowly with great tension until you reach full extension (see photo #3). Return to the starting position and continue. This can also be done from behind. Use slow, concentrated tension.

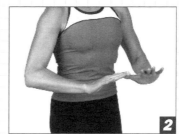
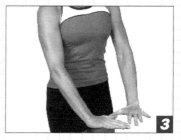

TR-9 (DSR)
FIST SALUTATION

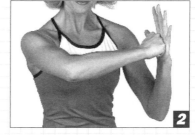

While this may look much like the Liederman Chest Press, it is distinct (see photo #1). Notice that your right fist is in your open left palm. The range of motion is from the right to the left. Switch hand positions to your left fist in your right palm and continue. 3 to 5 full range reps is all that is necessary. And, yes, I know you feel it in your pecs, too.

REPETITIONS	
MODERATE	10
HEAVY	6-8
VERY HEAVY	3-5

TR-10 (DVR)

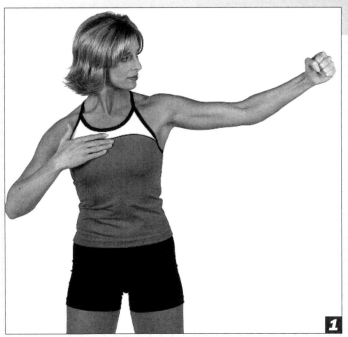
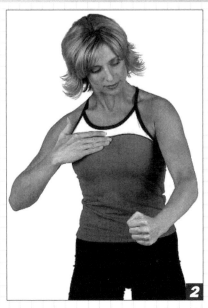
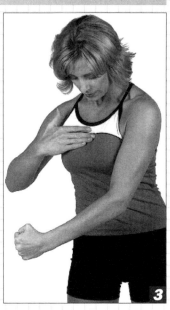

Stand with your feet at shoulder-width apart and your right hand fingers touching your sternum. Extend your left arm to eye level. Clench fist as tight as possible and powerfully flex biceps and triceps with as much tension as possible. (photo #1) Now slowly extend your left hand down and across to your upper right thigh while the muscles of the entire left arm are powerfully contracted. (photos #2-3) (This and all DVR exercises will feel as though you are moving with the brakes on.) Return to eye level while maintaining maximum tension. Do 3 to 5 ultra high tension reps and then switch sides and do 3 to 5 ultra high tension reps with your right arm.

TR-11 (DVR)
TRICEPS PRESS-DOWN

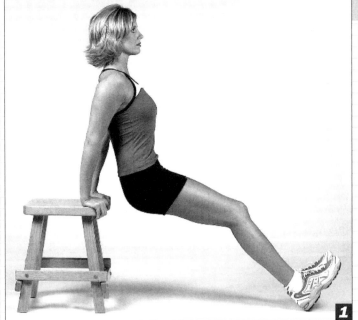
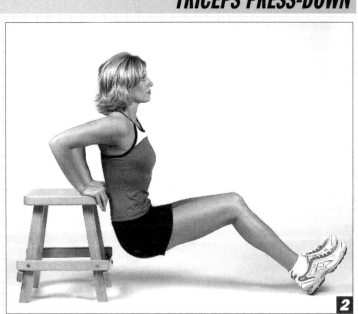

You may use a chair or stool for this exercise. Start with arms in a close to locked position, slowly lower your body as far as you can, then push back up to the starting position. Remember to use resistence through entire exercise.

LESSON TEN

every
WOMAN'S
GUIDE *to* **PERSONAL**
POWER

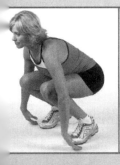
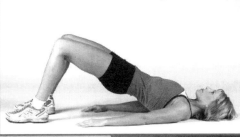
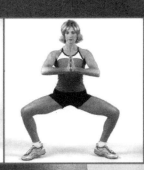

Thighs and Hamstrings

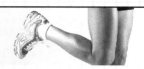

Okay, I know what you're probably thinking—this chapter is thicker than the rest. So why do I offer over 25 exercises for the legs while other sections have been limited to 10 to 15 exercises? The answer is simple. I know that most women suffer with trouble zones from their waist down, and I felt compelled to show you *all* the exercises I use for my legs and gluts. Keep in mind that I am repeating the Furey Push-up and the Furey Squat in this chapter as both of these exercises are absolutely incredible for the entire lower region of the body. The Furey Push-up is especially effective for your entire muscular system. You may adopt whichever exercises you feel most comfortable with and add intensity when you feel ready.

Once you get familiar with these exercises, you can actually do them throughout the day. For instance, when I curl my hair in the morning, I usually do a squat, plie, or hamstring curl with every curl of my hair. If I am waiting for water to boil in the kitchen, I squeeze in a few other *Transformetrics*™ leg moves. You get the picture. You can do *Transformetrics*™ moves throughout your busy day and start to enjoy the results.

Transformetrics™ will reduce any cellulite you may have lingering in the lower region of your body (or anywhere else for that matter). Over 90 percent of women have some type of cellulite on their thighs, hamstrings, and buttocks—even women in phenomenal shape. Why? Heredity and eating a diet high in fat are the usual suspects, but cellulite also deposits in this region as nature's way to get a woman's body ready to have children as it actually protects the unborn child. It's a simple fact of female life. It's not something that any of us are excited about, but it's nice to know that *Transformetrics*™ can help minimize the "cottage cheese" dilemma.

The goal of this chapter is simple—full, toned muscles, low overall body fat, a small waist, and control over the female tendency to store fat in the hips, thighs, and buttocks. Every exercise I show you will take you where you want to go.

Let's move ahead to the exercises that can help you go from lumpy to smooth, skinny to shapely, chunky to sleek in only a short amount of time.

TH-1 (PC)
THE FUREY PUSH-UP

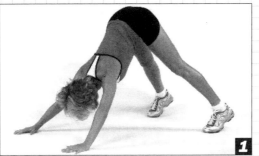
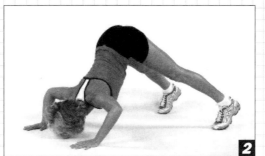

Photo #1. Start with your hands on the floor, shoulder-width apart, and your head tucked in and looking directly at your feet. Your feet are shoulder-width apart or slightly wider. Your legs and back are straight, and your butt is the highest point of the body.

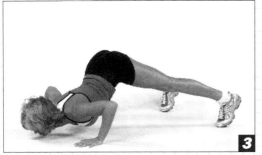
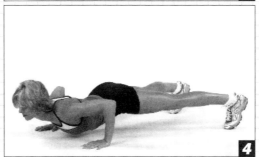

Photos #2-3-4-5. Bend your elbows while descending in a smooth circular arc almost brushing your chest and upper body to the floor as you continue the circular range of motion until your arms are straight, back flexed, and hips almost, but not quite, touching the floor.

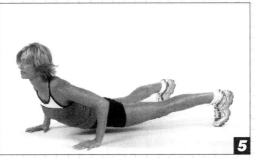
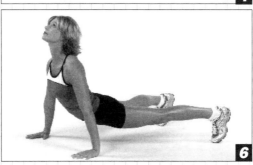

Photo #6. At the top of the movement, look at the ceiling while consciously flexing your triceps and exhaling.

Photo #7. Raise your hips and buttocks while simultaneously pushing back with straight arms, causing a complete articulation of both shoulder joints.

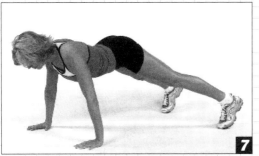
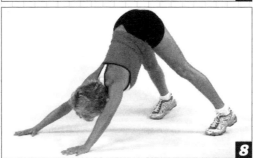

Photo #8. Arrive at the starting position with your legs and back straight, your head tucked in, and eyes looking at your feet.

Continue as smoothly and as fluidly as possible for as many repetitions as you can do.

At the beginning, anywhere from 15 to 25 repetitions is excellent. Once you can routinely do sets of 25 to 50 or more, you will have superb shoulder, chest, arm, and both upper and lower back development.

In my opinion this is the single greatest exercise. Repetition for repetition it delivers the highest level of strength, flexibility, and endurance of any calisthenic exercise known. In fact, it is the one exercise that comes closest to duplicating the exact movement of large jungle cats. It is truly one magnificent exercise.

TH-2 (PC)
THE FUREY SQUAT

This exercise is an amazing calisthenic. I do this exercise often, as it is a great cardiovascular move when done in high repetitions.

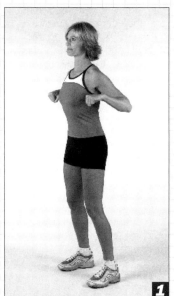
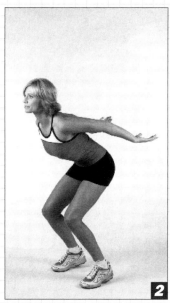
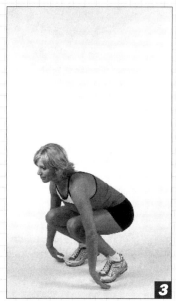

Photo #1. Feet approximately shoulder-width apart. Toes straight ahead. Hands in tight fists at shoulder level. Inhale deeply.

Photo #2. While keeping your back relatively straight (don't bend forward), bend your knees and descend to the bottom position.

Photo #3. Note the position of the hands reaching behind your back during the descent and brushing your knuckles on the ground at the bottom (how's that for a knuckle dragger?).

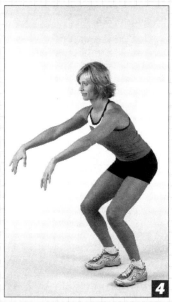
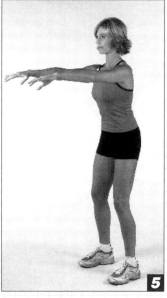
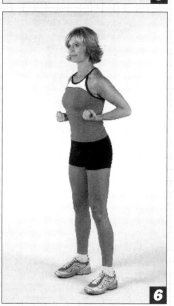

Photo #4. When you arrive at the bottom position, you will rise naturally to your toes. This is superb for your balance.

Photo #5. At this point your arms continue swinging forward and upward while simultaneously pushing off your toes and rising to the original standing position.

Photo #6. Your hands now form tight fists close to your sides at chest level. Inhale as you pull them in, exhale as you lower your body.

Repeat as smoothly and steadily as you can. Once you begin you'll notice that the arms take on a smooth, rhythmic motion similar to rowing a boat.

The entire movement of steps 1 to 6 is one continuous, smooth movement. 25 to 50 repetitions is a great start. 100 without stopping is excellent. Once you can do 350 or more in 20 minutes or less, you have accomplished the world's preeminent cardiovascular workout, not to mention a superb upper and lower leg workout. *Be careful. You may not be able to walk the next day!*

TH-3 (DSR)
LEG BICEPS CONTRACTION

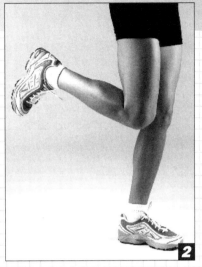

Study the photos carefully. While standing on your left leg, slowly bend your right leg at the knee and raise your right heel as close as possible to your right buttocks. Contract powerfully for a count of "one thousand one, one thousand two." Then straighten out your leg until you are standing on both feet again. Continue 3 to 5 high tension repetitions and do an Isometric Contraction on the last repetition only. Switch legs and continue.

TH-4 (ISO)
WALL SQUAT AND HOLD

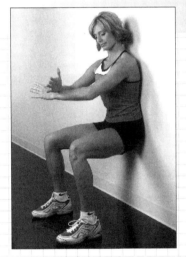

Stand with your feet approximately 20" from the wall. Slowly lower your body into a parallel squat. Your back should be touching the wall. Once you reach the parallel position you will hold as long as you can—up to 3 minutes. Yes, the muscles will shake. One repetition only.

TH-5 (DSR)
LEG EXTENSION

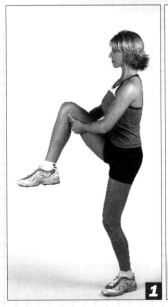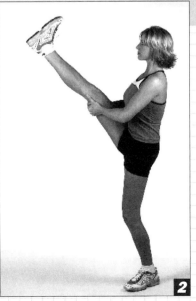

While standing on your left leg, raise your right leg to the position shown with your knee bent, toes pointed. Slowly, with great concentration, extend your right leg, endeavoring to fully extend and straighten it. 3 to 5 reps max. Switch legs and repeat.

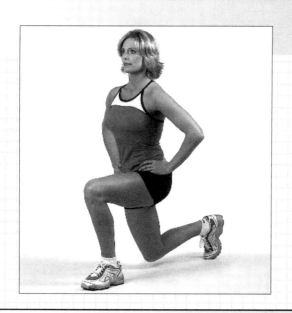

TH-6 (PC)
LUNGES

Hands on hips. Take a step forward while bending the left knee and lowering yourself until your outstretched right knee barely touches the floor. Keep your left knee above your ankle as you bend very slowly, using your left quadriceps to control the motion up and down. Complete 3 to 5 high-tension repetitions (more if you want). Switch the relative position of the legs and repeat.

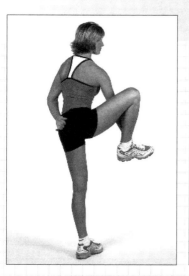 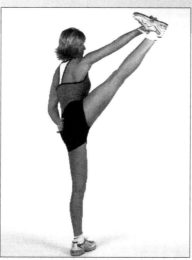

TH-7 (DSR)
LIEDERMAN LEG PRESS OUT

See the photos. This one looks odd and is not easy. Grasp your right heel with your right hand and raise your leg as high as you possibly can, extending against the resistance of your right hand until your knee is straight. It's the last part, the straightening of the knee that is most difficult. Do 3 to 5 intense reps with both legs (more if you want). This exercise develops the leg biceps.

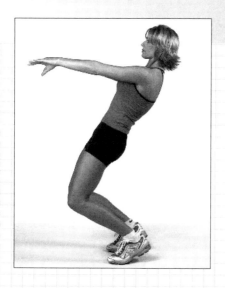

TH-8 (PC)
SISSY SQUAT

I don't have a clue as to who named this exercise, but you don't have to be a pansy to do it! Have your feet about 12" apart and hands outstretched or on hips to keep your balance (see photo). Slowly lower your body by squatting down. Maintain the hips forward position throughout the exercise. Raise and lower slowly. 12 to 20 reps is great.

TH-9 (PC)
KARATE KICK-OUT

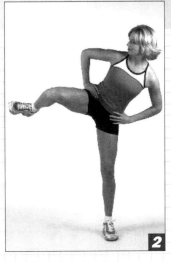
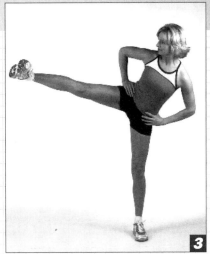

Bring right leg up in a side hinge to prepare for a kick and follow through to extend leg fully. Use maximum tension. Repeat with other leg.

TH-10 (PC)
HAMSTRING PRESS OUT

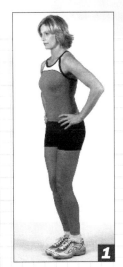
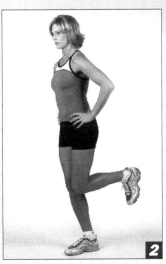
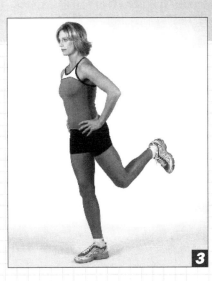

Start with your legs together and raise your left leg while fully contracting your hamstring, then press out as if pushing against a wall with your foot. Return your extended leg to the other leg and then back to starting position. Reverse with other leg. Great for hamstrings and gluts.

TH-11 (PC)
HINGE

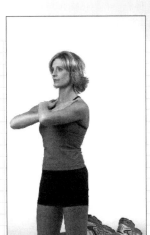
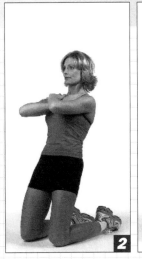
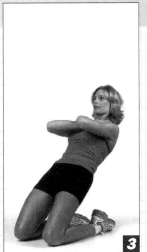

Start on your knees with arms crossed over chest. Hinge back while contracting thighs, gluts, and abs.

TH-12 (DVR)
DONKEY KICK

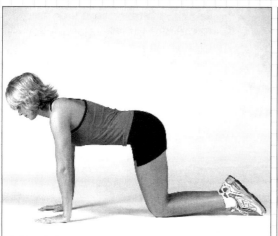 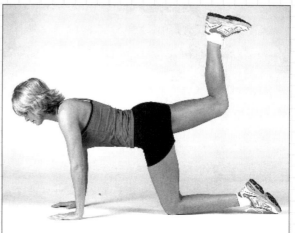

In the table top position, lift right leg while flexing hamstrings and gluts. Raise your foot to the ceiling. Press up in a slow controlled pulsing action. Reverse and repeat with left leg.

TH-13 (DVR)
SIDE HINGE W/BACK EXTENSION

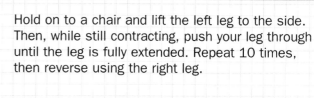

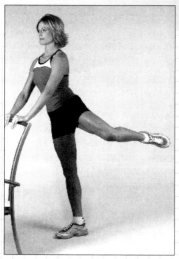 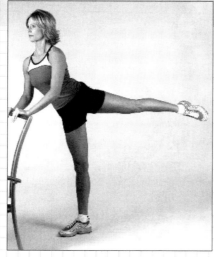

Hold on to a chair and lift the left leg to the side. Then, while still contracting, push your leg through until the leg is fully extended. Repeat 10 times, then reverse using the right leg.

TH-14 (PC)
LUNGE W/TRUNK ROTATION

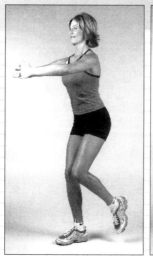 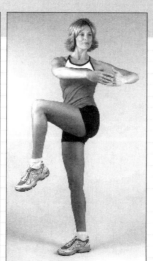

Start in a right lunge position. (Remember to keep you front leg in a 90° angle—do not extend over your toes.) Use hip and thigh muscles to straighten legs, and bring left knee through and forward up to hip height, simultaneously circling arms to left side and twisting torso to the left. Return to starting position and repeat.

TH-15 (PC)
PREP KICK OUT

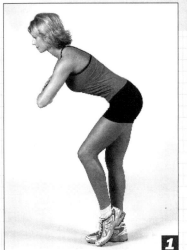
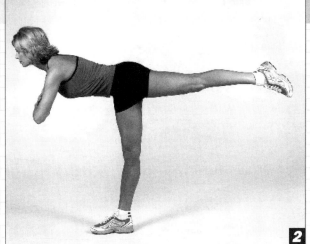

Prep with your left leg. With hip and thigh muscles extend your left leg behind you until body forms a straight line from heel to head. Hold with tension. Slowly lower your foot to starting position and repeat. Switch legs and repeat process. Great for lower back, gluts, thighs, hamstrings, and abs.

TH-16 (PC)
THE SKATE

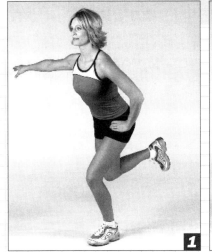
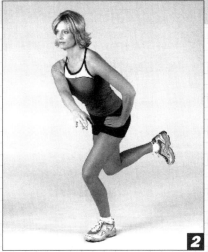

Photo #1. Stand on left leg, lift right foot behind body, knee bent, hands on hips. Leaning forward, squat (keep knee over foot) and extend right arm to right. Return to start.

Photo #2. Repeat, reaching in a different direction with each squat for a balance challenge. Finish reps on left leg. Then switch legs and repeat. Great for gluts, thighs, and abs.

TH-17 (PC)
LIFT, REACH, AND STRETCH

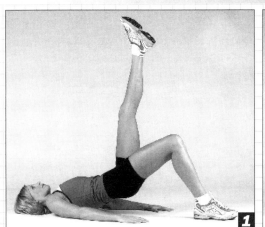
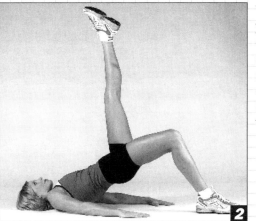

While lying on your back, bend your right leg keeping your foot on the floor. Raise your left leg straight up to the ceiling, then push up using the hamstrings, quads, and abs. This doesn't have to be a huge movement to be effective.

TH-18 (DVR)
LIFT W/KEGEL

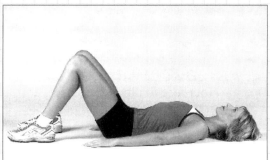 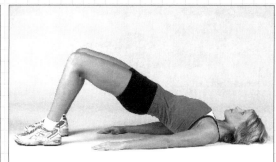

Lie down and bend both legs keeping both feet on floor. Then press up with your hips as far as possible with a Kegel contraction for 5 to 10 seconds. This exercise is very important for women to practice routinely.

TH-19 (PC)
STANDARD SQUAT

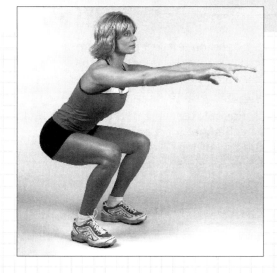

Squat by sitting back and keeping weight into heels. Remember, your knees should not bend over the toes as this causes stress on the knee itself. (You may add a bicep/tricep curl to this move.)

TH-20 (PC)
ONE-LEGGED SQUAT W/TOWEL

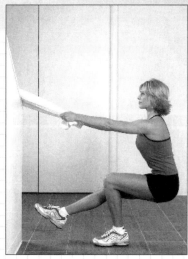

Using a towel wrapped around a permanent object, grab each end. While resisting your weight, slowly lower into a one-legged squat. Return to start position and repeat.

TH-21 (PC/DSR)
BALANCE SQUAT W/C'MON AT YA!

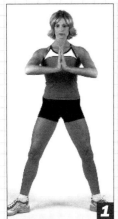 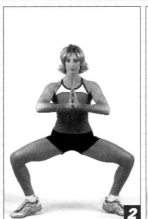 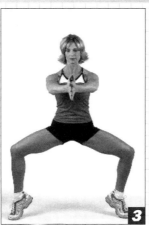 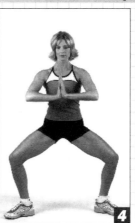

Stand with feet slightly wider than shoulder-width apart, toes turned out and hands in prayer position. Pull navel into spine. Keeping back straight, bend knees into a squat until thighs are almost parallel to the ground. Arch up high on toes to strengthen calves and practice balance. At the same time, perform the C'Mon At Ya series with upper body.

TH-22 (DVR)
PRONE LEG KICK

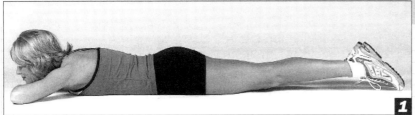

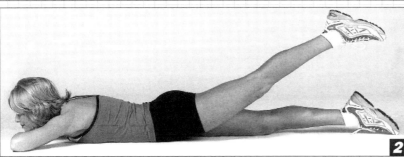

Lie face down on the ground, resting chin on hands. Keeping hips on the ground, slowly raise your left leg. Return to start. Repeat, alternating legs.

TH-23 (DVR)
WALKING HALF-BEND

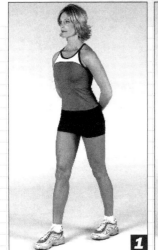 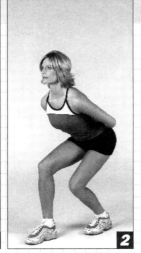

With one foot 8" to 10" in front of the other, bend while contracting thigh and glut muscles.

TH-24 (PC)
SIDE HINGE

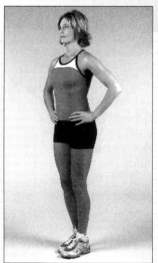 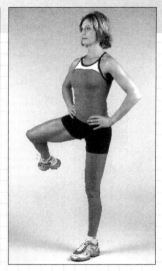

Start with legs together and lift right leg hinging at the hip. Make sure to contract gluts and thighs.

TH-25 (PC)
REVERSE LUNGE W/LEG EXTENSION

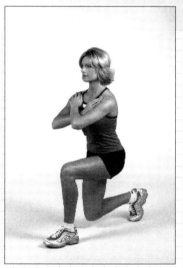 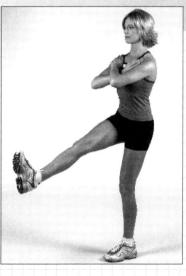

Step back with your right leg into a lunge position, keeping torso erect. Using your gluts and thigh muscles, straighten your left leg and bring your right knee forward to just below hip height. Without leaning back, use your thigh muscles to straighten your leg. Hold for five counts before returning to the starting position. Repeat, then switch legs.

Question & Answer

Q: During my menstrual cycle I get super tired and unmotivated. Any suggestions?

A: I would like to suggest you consider using Revival Soy products. Countless testimonials have shown that soy can increase energy levels during this time along with reducing any cramping that may go along with PMS. The motivation part is entirely up to you, of course! But with energy and a sense of not feeling miserable, it helps matters tremendously. See page 55 for more information on Revival Soy.

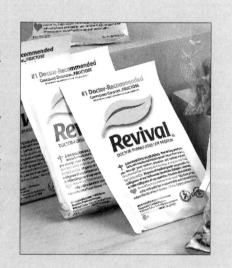

LESSON ELEVEN

every
WOMAN'S
GUIDE *to* **PERSONAL**
POWER

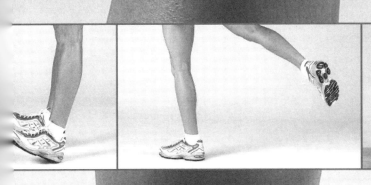
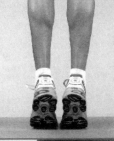

Calves

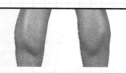

Ah, the icing on the cake for shapely legs. Calves complete the overall look of healthy, fit legs. Perhaps you're among the lucky few who don't have to work very hard to have sculpted calves. Chalk that up to your genetics. For most of us, to build and shape our calves requires some serious assistance. I am pleased to offer you several exercises that will make a world of difference.

Based on my past experience I want to caution you to gradually work up to added tension and repetitions with these exercises as the soreness will sneak up on you if you do not. It's not what I call a fun morning when you hop out of bed and fall straight to the floor in pain due to overworking your calves. And then you crawl...literally crawl...to the bathroom. This happened to me when I first started *Transformetrics*™ and was doing calf raises in the living room while watching *Fear Factor* on television. I was so caught up in all the gross events going on—anything from slimy worm eating contests to people climbing into a glass box full of tarantulas only to allow them to crawl all over them. Thinking about that again gives me the heebie-jeebies. Anyway, I totally lost track of how long I had performed the calve raises, and at the time my calves weren't sore, just seriously pumped.

Moral to this story: pay attention to what you are doing or you'll pay attention the following morning!

These calve exercises will not only help you sculpt and tone, but they will assist you in overall balance, which is important and should go hand-in-hand with strength and endurance training. You will find these exercises as easy or challenging as you make them.

CV-1

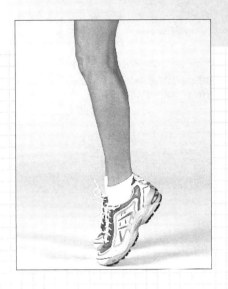

Stand with one foot a little in front of the other. Slowly rise as high as possible on your toes, trying to stand on the tip of the tip. (Hey, I said try. I'm not expecting you to be a ballerina.)

CV-2

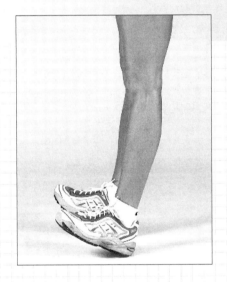

Stand with your feet 18" to 24" apart and support the weight of your body on the heels with the toes turned outward. Build the tension and hold for a "one thousand one, one thousand two." Then switch positions. Support your weight on your toes with your heels turned outward. Now slowly reverse it again. You'll notice that your feet come closer together with each repetition. Make sure you can consciously stretch and contract the muscles as much as possible.

CV-3

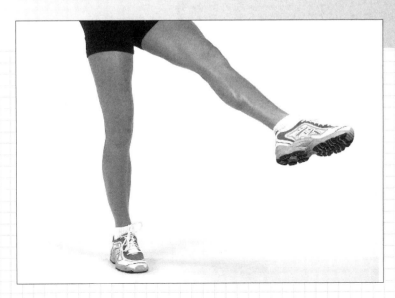

While standing on your right foot, raise your left foot from the floor and stretch it out as far as you can while pointing the toes downward. Switch legs and repeat. Contract the calf muscle powerfully, but go easy at first or you may get a charley horse.

CV-4

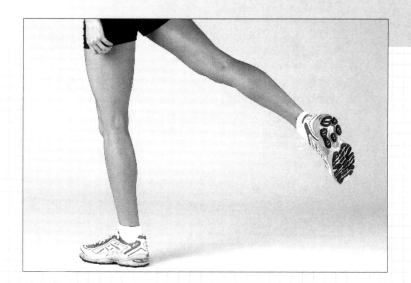

Same exercise as CV-3 except that your leg is stretched behind the body. Follow the same procedure and then switch legs.

CV-5

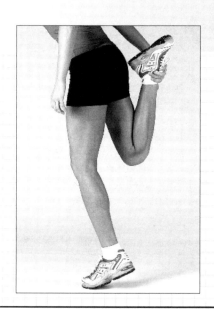

Rise up on your left foot as shown in the photos. You may hold on to the other foot. Slowly but powerfully contract the muscles. Yes, this is tougher than it looks.

CV-6

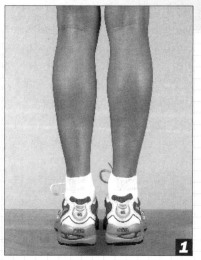
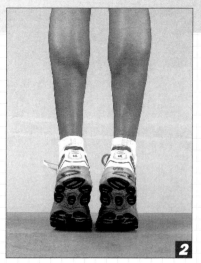

While standing with the ball of the foot on the edge of a chair, a step, or a thick telephone directory, rise on the toes as high as is convenient. Slowly and powerfully contract the calf muscles. Hold the peak contraction for "one thousand one, one thousand two."

CV-7

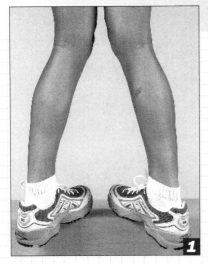 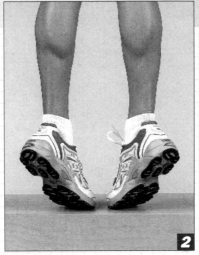

While standing with toes together and heels apart on the edge of a chair, a step, or a thick telephone directory, rise on the toes as high as is convenient. Slowly and powerfully contract the calf muscles. Hold the peak contraction for "one thousand one, one thousand two."

CV-8

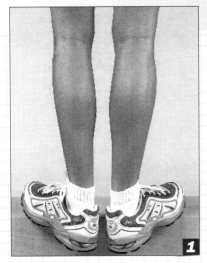 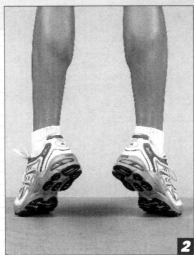

While standing with heels together and toes apart on the edge of a chair, a step, or a thick telephone directory, rise on the toes as high as is convenient. Slowly and powerfully contract the calf muscles. Hold the peak contraction for "one thousand one, one thousand two."

Question & Answer

Q: I noticed that you offer more lower body exercises than in any other section. Is there a reason for this?

A: Most women I have ever known are more concerned about their shape from the waist down. I offer over 40 exercises for abs and legs so you have several to interchange with and break up the monotony. They are all incredibly effective, and some can be very challenging based on the tension involved. One of my personal favorites is the Furey Squat.

Question & Answer

Q: I am 35 pounds overweight and want to shed these pounds before my upcoming 20-year class reunion. How much cardio should I be doing weekly?

A: This is a great question, although the answer could vary for every individual. First of all, it depends on the amount of training time you have prior to your reunion. If say you have anywhere from 4 to 6 months, I would put you on a program of 30 to 45 minutes of cardio, three times a week. But you need to do the *Transformetrics*™ exercises daily to replace the weight that is lost with lean muscle. Believe me, everyone will be in awe when they see you at the reunion and want to know your secrets!

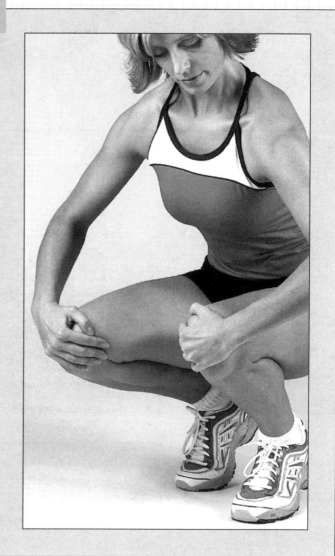

LESSON TWELVE

Power Calisthenics

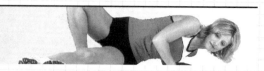

Calisthenics require balancing and stabilizing muscles, which act together in real-life situations to coordinate movement. This optimizes the development of overall body strength. I consider power calisthenics to be functional exercises (movements that mimic everyday or sports movements) and make the most sense for practical strength. For example, these multiple-joint exercises involve pushing, pulling, and squatting and provide crossover benefit for many activities. They train your muscles the way they will be used.

Many athletes become superior ones because they use their whole body as a training workout tool. In many cases it is not how strong and powerful the athlete is but how he or she best uses his or her strength and power that determines athletic success. When athletes train with calisthenics that incorporate many muscles, tendons, ligaments, and bones in a natural progression, they are better prepared to use their whole body in sports skills. It is of utmost importance that an athlete's (or an aspiring one's) strength training incorporate the use of the whole body.

Transformetrics™ provides a quick, safe workout for the beginner as well as the most advanced athlete. However, for the beginner the power calisthenics may prove to be integrated best once you have been on the program for a while. The calisthenics I show are not out of reach for many women, but some of you will need to build your strength and endurance before you are able to master these. You have already been introduced to the most essential power calisthenics: the Furey Push-up, the Furey Squat, the Atlas Push-up, and the Furey Bridge. These four exercises alone will help you achieve true dynamic athletic fitness and super health.

Once you start truly connecting with the power calisthenics, you'll realize that it's not the number of reps of a certain exercise you can do but the overall quality and awareness you achieve between your mind and your muscles that counts. Your numbers will increase gradually when your body is ready and able. Don't get hung up on the numbers game. Remember: everyone is different and can accomplish different goals due to their somatotypes or God-given shape. For example, someone with long arms will typically have a harder time doing pull-ups then someone with short arms, because the range is much farther to reach the top of the pull-up.

My main advice, not only during power calisthenics but throughout this book, is to listen to what your body tells you that you can and can't do. It takes patience, but eventually your body will arrive at where your mind is wanting to go. You are here to learn and practice these exercises to the best of your ability. No one will judge you by your learning curve or individual feats of strength. Do what you can and know that you are a true athlete at your own level.

GROUP I: NECK
1. FUREY BRIDGE

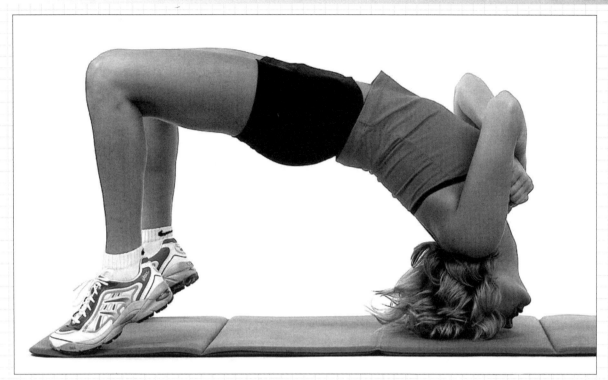

GROUP I:
2. REVERSE FUREY BRIDGE & LADIES BRIDGE

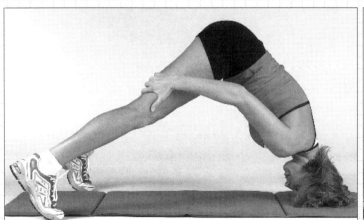

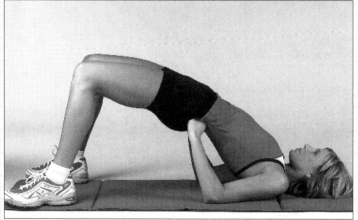

Work up to their performance very gradually and if you feel any pain—STOP! They are both very advanced exercises and require the utmost of care and caution when performing either one.

LADIES BRIDGE: This bridge is a great modification of the Furey Bridge. It allows for an amazing stretch in the lower back.

GROUP II:
SHOULDERS, CHEST, TRICEPS, UPPER BACK, & ABS
1. FUREY PUSH-UP

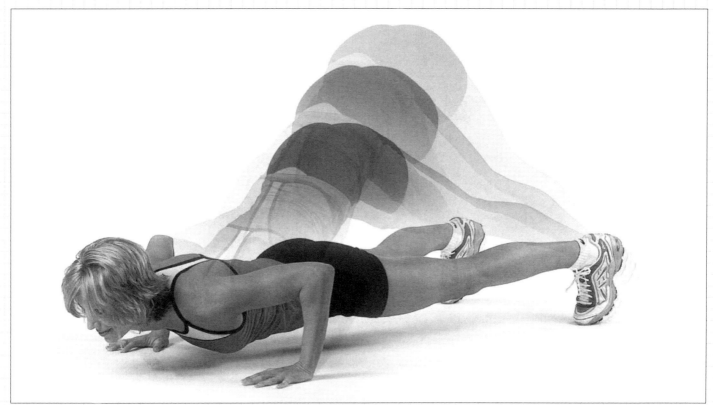

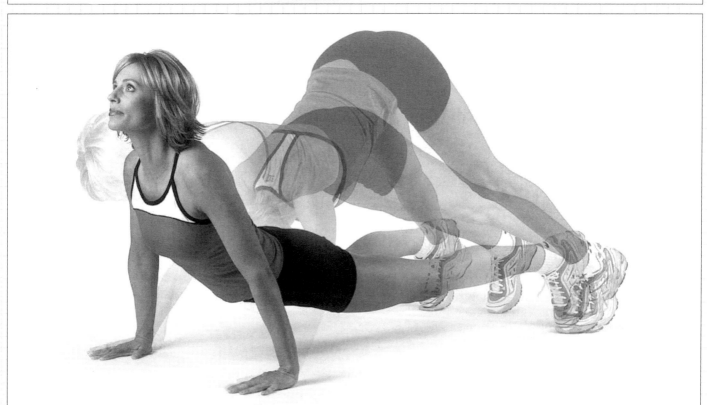

See page 46 for complete instructions.

GROUP II:
2. STANDARD LIEDERMAN PUSH-UP

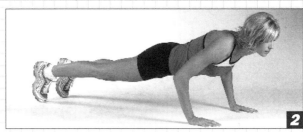

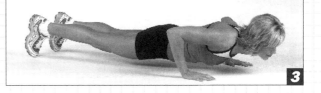

GROUP II:
3. LIEDERMAN PUSH-UP (VARIATION)

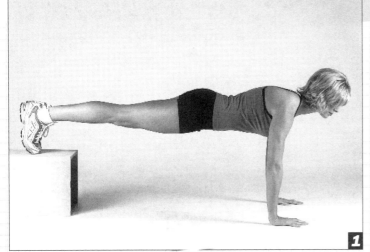

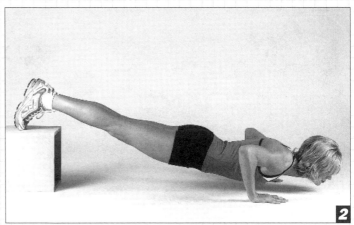

GROUP II:
4. STANDARD ATLAS PUSH-UP

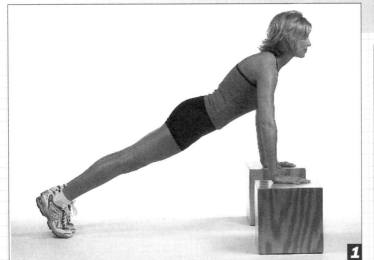

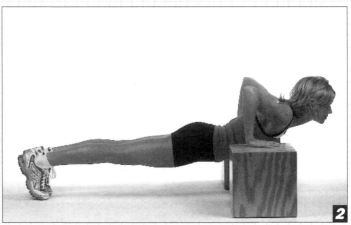

GROUP II:
5. ATLAS PUSH-UP (VARIATION)

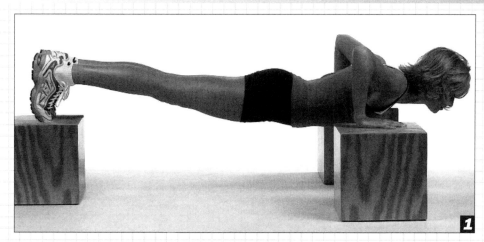

GROUP II:
6. TRICEPS PUSH-UP

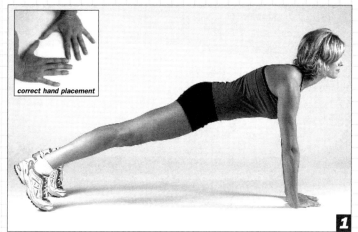

correct hand placement

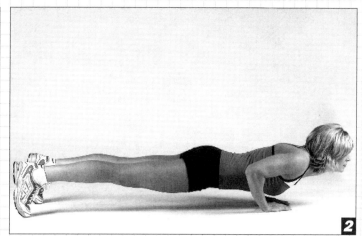

GROUP II:
7. ONE-LEGGED PUSH-UP

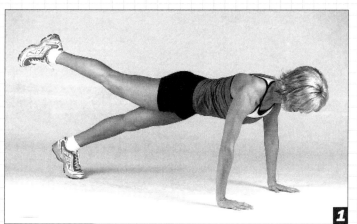

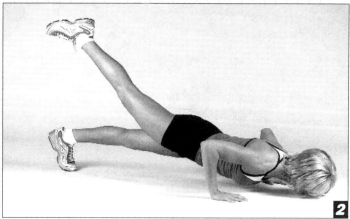

GROUP II:
8. MODIFIED PUSH-UP

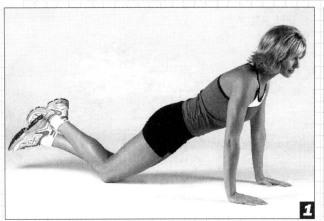
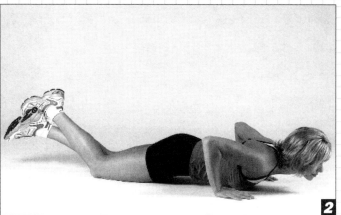

GROUP II:
9. HANDSTAND PUSH-UP

These are a little scary at first, but with the wall to kick up to you will become more at ease. Once you can perform a few handstand push-ups, then I would say you are truly strong and probably a great athlete. Don't try these prior to warming up.

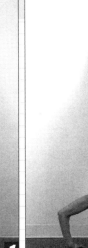
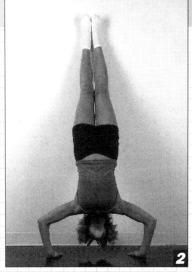

GROUP II:
10. SIDE PUSH-UP W/INNER THIGH LEG RAISE

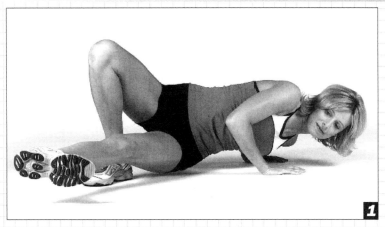

Place left hand on floor and swing left leg forward so right thigh and calf hover the floor, keeping the foot flexed. Place right hand on floor and bend elbows to lower left ear and chest close to floor. Torso and left leg should form a right angle. While holding here, pulse left leg for 15 to 20 reps. Repeat exercise on opposite side. Great for inner thighs, obliques, and arms.

Advanced Version: Perform side push-up in conjunction with leg raises.

GROUP III: BACK, BICEPS, & FOREARMS

1. WIDE GRIP PULL-UP

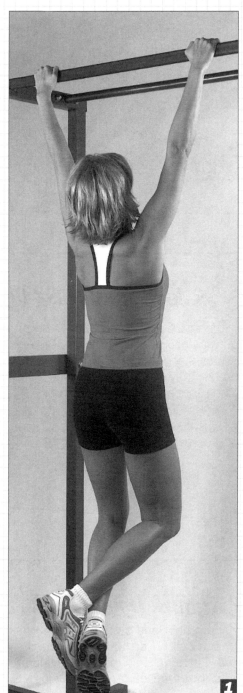
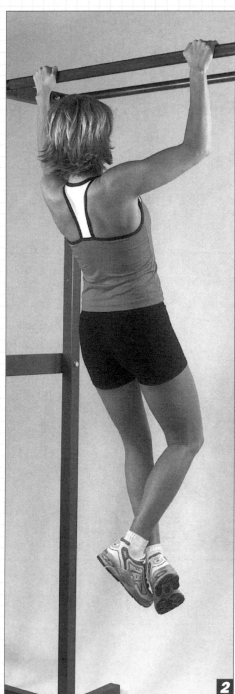
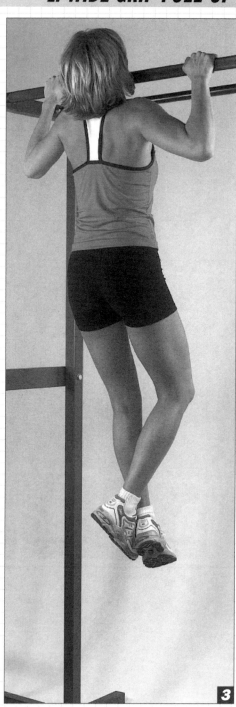

Please Note:

1. **ALL PULL-UPS** are performed with palms facing away from the body.

2. **ALL CHIN-UPS** are performed with palms facing the body.

This represents the distinction between a pull-up and a chin-up.

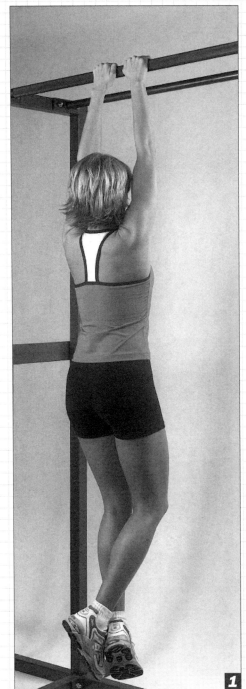
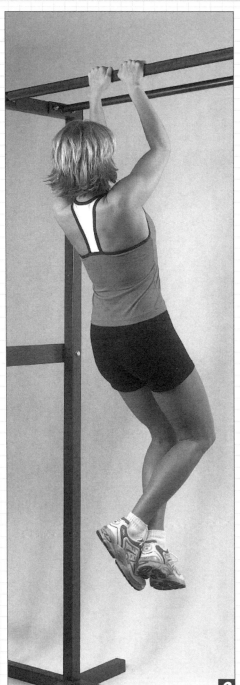
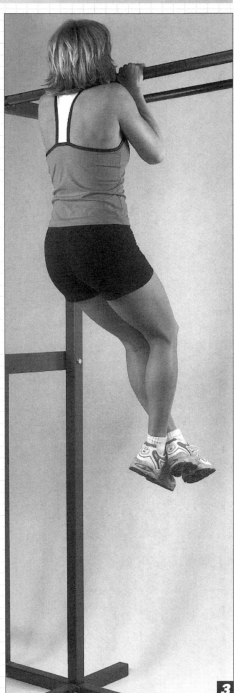

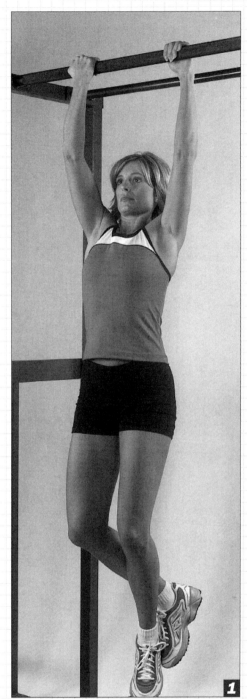

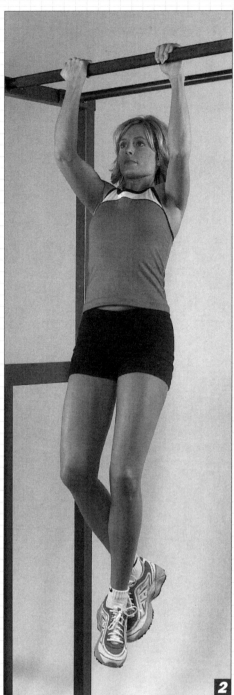

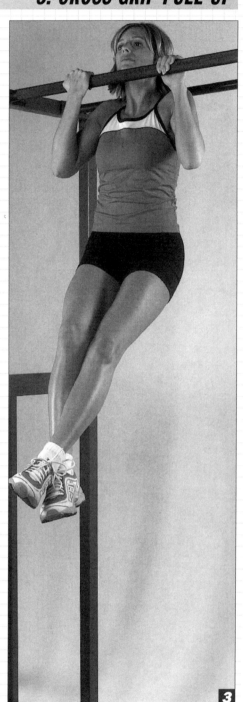

GROUP IV: ABDOMINALS
1. ATLAS SIT-UP

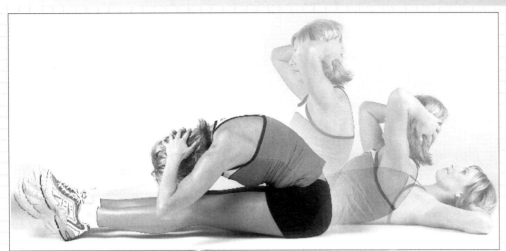

Anybody who says sit-ups don't work your abs has obviously never done Atlas Sit-ups. Done full-range, your forehead or chin should touch your knees on each repetition. The secret is that the feet are *not* held down. It is muscle contraction alone that keeps them down. That is why this exercise works incredibly well. However, both this and the Atlas Leg Raise (Group IV #2) should only be done to your present range of motion. **So be careful.**

GROUP IV:
2. ATLAS LEG RAISE

Full range dynamic flexibility

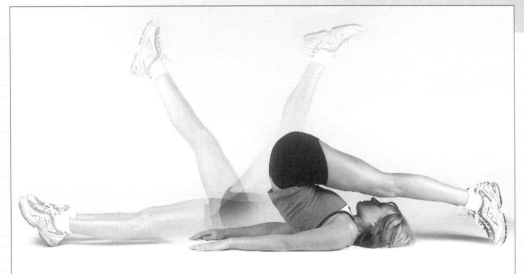

GROUP IV:
3. ATLAS COMBINATION

Strength, coordination, balance

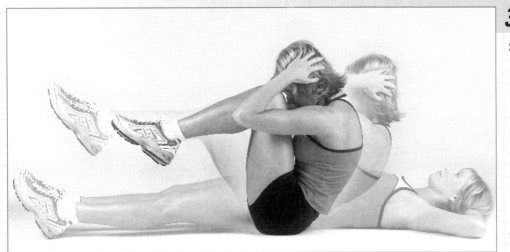

GROUP IV:
4. V-UPS

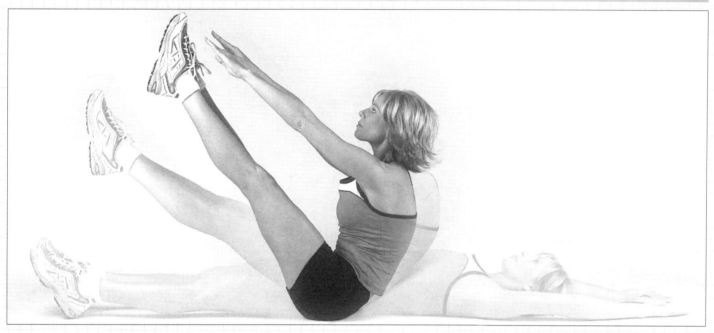

Strength, coordination, balance

GROUP IV:
5. SUPERWOMAN — WHEEL

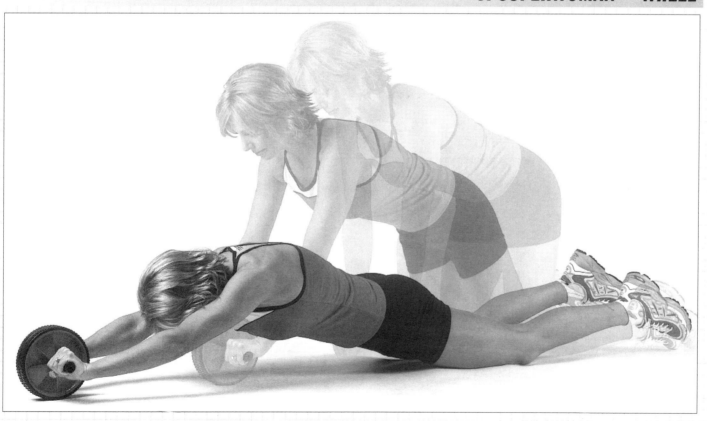

GROUP V: UPPER LEGS
1. FUREY SQUAT

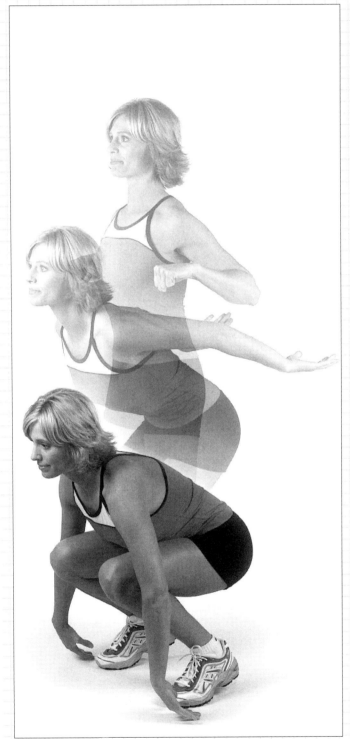

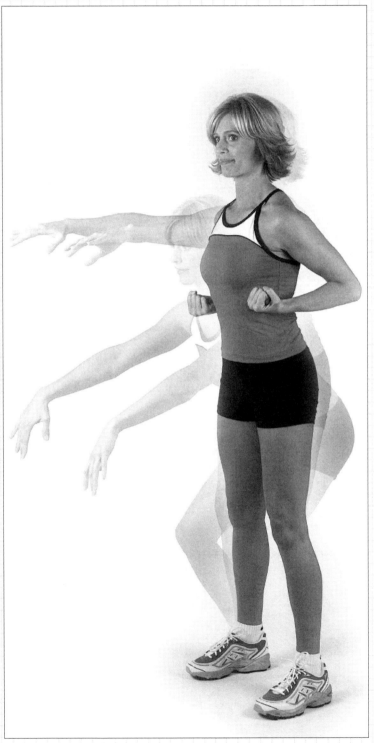

See page 49 for complete instructions.

GROUP V:
2. LEG EXTENSION

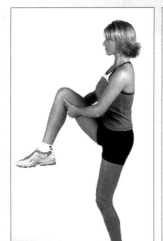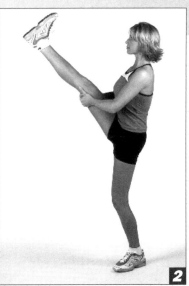

GROUP V:
3. LUNGE

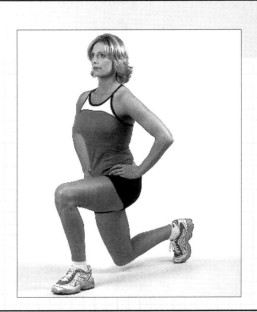

GROUP V:
4. SISSY SQUAT

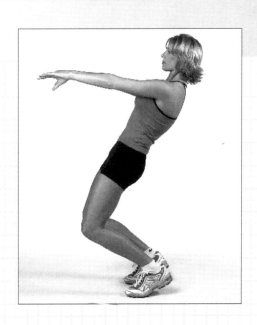

GROUP V:
5. HIGH KICK (FRONT, BACK, SIDE)

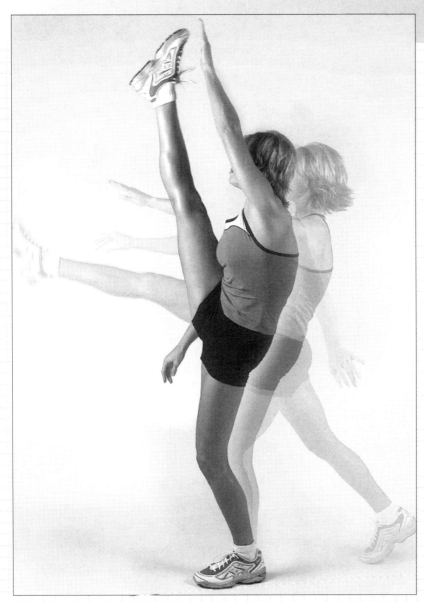

GROUP V:
6. PLANK JUMP-SQUAT

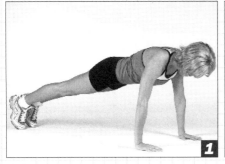 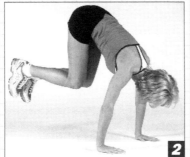 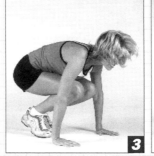 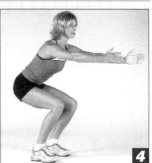

Start in plank position, hands under shoulders, feet and legs together, abs tight. Next jump forward, landing feet outside hands. Rise to a squat, arms extended. Return to plank. Works chest, arms, abs, thighs, and gluts.

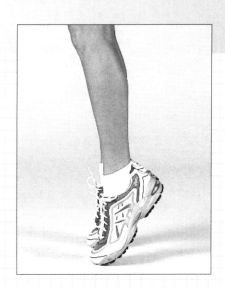

GROUP VI: CALVES
1. TOE RAISES

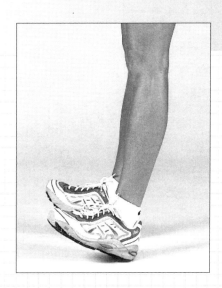

GROUP VI:
2. HEEL RAISES

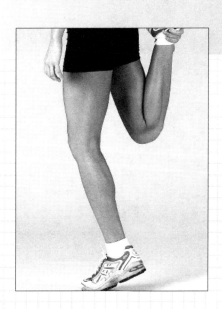

GROUP VI:
3. SINGLE LEG TOE RAISE

GROUP VI:
4. TOE RAISE OFF BOX

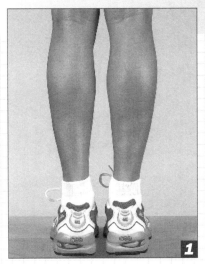 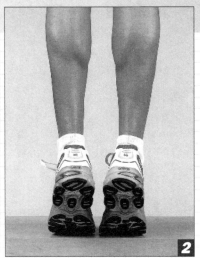

GROUP VI:
5. PIGEON TOE RAISE OFF BOX

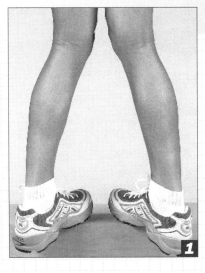 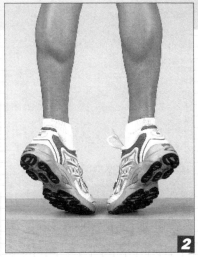

GROUP VI:
6. DUCK TOE RAISE OFF BOX

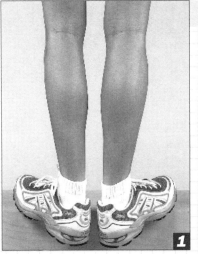 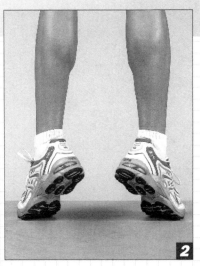

Hotline Numbers and Web Sites
FOR WOMEN IN NEED OF ASSISTANCE

ANAD—National Association of Anorexia Nervosa and Associate Disorders: www.anad.org and 847.831.3438

ANRED—Anorexia Nervosa and Related Eating Disorders: www.anred.com

Bulimia and Self-help Hotline (24-hour crisis line): 314.588.1683

EDAP—National Eating Disorders Awareness and Prevention: www.edap.org and www.nationaleatingdisorders.org and 800.931.2237

Overeaters Anonymous: www.oa.org and 505.891.2664

The Renfrew Center—for all eating disorders: www.renfrew.org and 800.736.3739

Something Fishy—Web Site on Eating Disorders: www.something-fishy.org

Eating Disorders Association in the United Kingdom:
Adult hotline: 0845.634.1414, Youthline: 0845.634.7650

The Eating Distress Helpline in Ireland: 01.2600366

My Personal Guarantee

You have now completed this book and have everything you need in order to begin to guide you into a new way of living. There is no excuse for not starting as I have demonstrated every exercise with photos and detailed instructions. I challenge you to start today!

I guarantee that all the exercises in this book have been tried and proven, and you will see results with every bit of increased strength. Every exercise I teach was in turn taught to me by John Peterson along with a few added exercises devoted to women and our targeted "tough zones." You will see results if you follow the exercises along with the nutrition guidelines.

GUARANTEED!

Let's get empowered. "You Go Girls." I am pulling for you through thick and thin.

You are all MY motivation.

Best always,

Wendie Pett

P.S. You can contact me through Bronze Bow Publishing at **www.bronzebowpublishing.com**. I'd like to hear from you and don't forget to send me your before and after photos.

"The Sovereign Lord has taught me what to say,
so that I can strengthen the weary."

—Isaiah 50:4

Notes

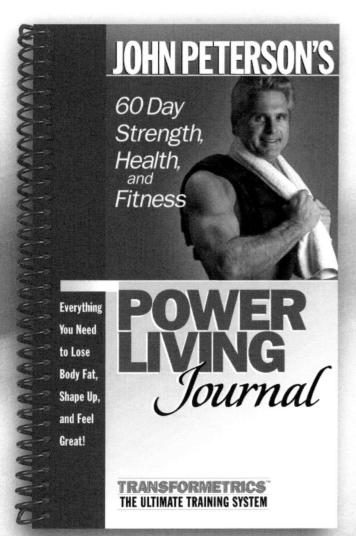

Power Living Journal
by John Peterson
ISBN 1-932458-16-6
(5 1/4 x 8 1/2)
Available: June 15, 2004

DESIGNED FOR *YOU* to **SUCCEED**

John's for the Men

Wendie's for the Ladies

Both offer the most honest, straightforward approach to safe, lifelong strength, youthfulness, and long-term fat loss you'll ever find.

Let's get real. There is no quick fix. There are no magic diets. And nobody has a magic wand to give you the lithe, athletic, sculpted physique or figure you've always dreamed of having. You need three things: the right balance of nutritious foods, the right strength-building, body-sculpting exercise system, and the knowledge and commitment to put them together.

In the *Power Living Journals*, John and Wendie offer you:

• A complete exercise program featuring the *Transformetrics™ Training System* requiring just minutes a day to help you slim, strengthen, and achieve your body's natural, God-given strength and fitness potential…without the requirement of a gym or expensive exercise equipment.

• Complete food charts that feature protein, fat, and carbohydrate grams as well as calories.

• User-friendly exercise charts to help you keep track of your daily progress.

• And inspiring quotes, scriptures, and more to help you stay motivated.

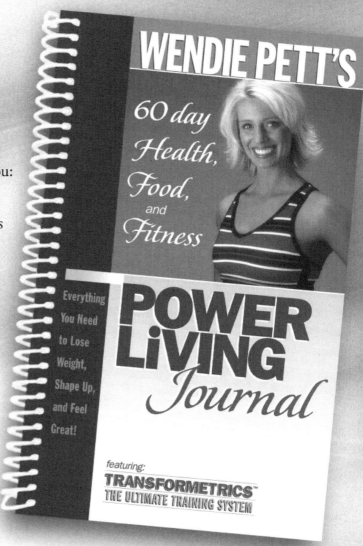

Power Living Journal
by Wendie Pett
ISBN 1-932458-15-8
(5 1/4 x 8 1/2)
Available: June 15, 2004

IF YOU'VE BEEN LOOKING FOR AN EXERCISE SYSTEM
that will give you the results you've always dreamed of having, does not require a gym or expensive exercise equipment, can be done anytime and anyplace without requiring an outrageous commitment of time, *this book is it.*

Based solidly upon the most effective exercise systems as taught by Earle E. Liederman and Charles Atlas during the 1920s, *Pushing Yourself to Power* provides you with everything you need to know to help your body achieve its natural, God-given strength and fitness potential. Whether your desire is simply to slim down and shape up, or to build your maximum all-around functional strength, athletic fitness, and *natural* muscularity, you will find complete training strategies specifically tailored to the achievement of your personal goals.

Profusely illustrated with 100s of clear, detailed photos showing every facet of every exercise, you'll never have to guess if you're doing it right again. You'll achieve the stamina you've always wanted in less time than it requires to drive to a gym and change into exercise clothes. Feel what it's like to have twice as much energy as you ever thought you'd have!

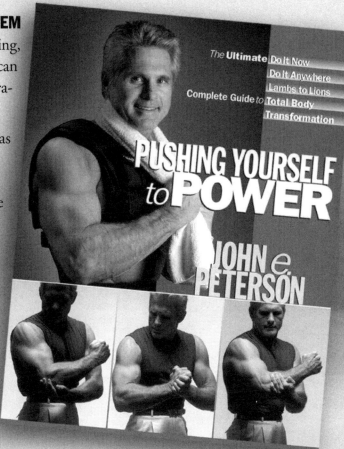

Pushing Yourself to Power
by John Peterson
ISBN 1-932458-01-8
Available in trade or spiral (8 1/2 x 11)

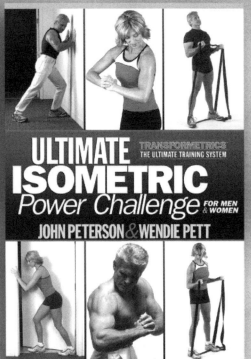

Ultimate Isometric Power Challenge
by John Peterson & Wendie Pett
ISBN 1-932458-11-5 (6 x 9)
Available: Spring 2004

"He trains my hands for battle; my arms can bend a bow of bronze."

In 2 Samuel 22:35 and Psalm 18:34, King David praises God for blessing him with his obvious strength. And though it may not be necessary for everyone to have King David's strength, wouldn't it be wonderful to have lifelong health, strength, energy, and a beautifully sculpted body?

featuring:
TRANSFORMETRICS™
THE ULTIMATE TRAINING SYSTEM

The good news is anyone can, and a lot sooner than he or she ever dreamed possible. At Bronze Bow we own the trademark for the Transformetrics™ Training System—the ultimate system for men and women to not only maximize their strength and fitness but to also sculpt their bodies to their own natural, God-given perfection. Best of all, Transformetrics™ requires no gym or equipment.

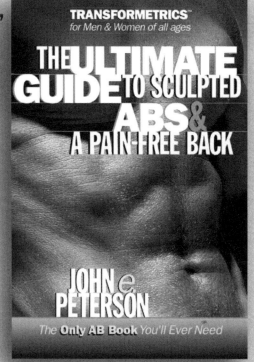

The Ultimate Guide to Sculpted Abs & a Pain-free Back
by John Peterson
ISBN 1-932458-12-3 (6 x 9)
Available: Spring 2004

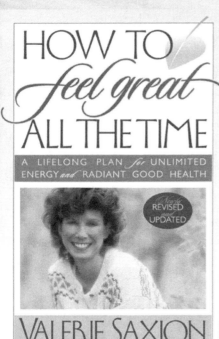

How to Feel Great All the Time

A lifelong plan for unlimited and radiant good health in four basic steps.

ISBN 0-9724563-5-X
$19.99 trade (5 3/8 x 8 1/4)

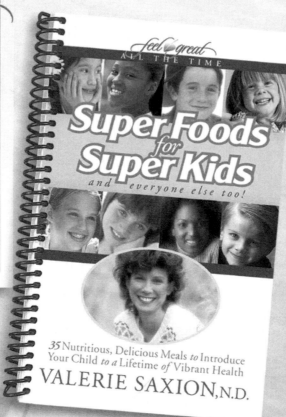

Super Foods for Super Kids

ISBN 1-932458-03-4
$19.99 spiral (5 3/8 x 8 1/4)

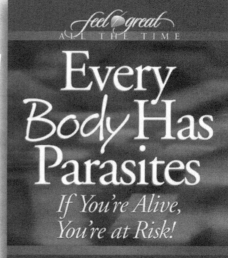

Every Body Has Parasites

Exposes the hidden crisis that is damaging millions of people needlessly today. A recent health report stated that 85 percent of Americans are infected with parasites.

ISBN 1-932458-00-X
$14.99 trade (5 3/8 x 8 1/4)

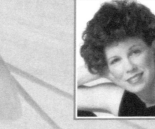

VALERIE SAXION

One of America's most articulate champions of nutrition and natural healing, Valerie is a twenty-year veteran of health science with a primary focus in naturopathy. She is the host of the weekly Trinity Broadcasting Network program *On Call* and is also seen regularly on Daystar Television Network and Cornerstone Television Networks.

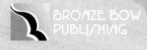

BRONZE BOW
PUBLISHING

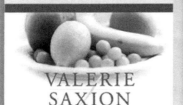

ISBN 0-9724563-7-6
$7.99 trade (4 1/2 x 7)

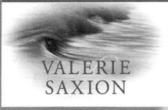

ISBN 0-9724563-8-4
$7.99 trade (4 1/2 x 7)

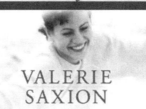

ISBN 0-9724563-9-2
$7.99 trade (4 1/2 x 7)

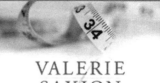

ISBN 0-9724563-6-8
$7.99 trade (4 1/2 x 7)

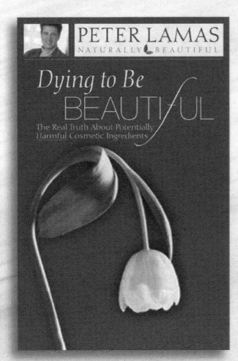

Health and Fitness Glossary

Peter's comprehensive guide to the complex terminology of the health and fitness world.

ISBN 1-932458-08-5
(5 3/8 x 8 1/4)
Available: Spring 2004

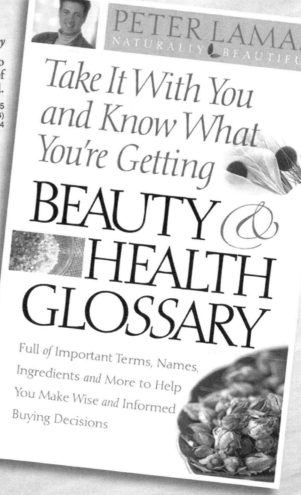

Take It With You and Know What You're Getting

BEAUTY & HEALTH GLOSSARY

Full of Important Terms, Names, Ingredients and More to Help You Make Wise and Informed Buying Decisions

Dying to Be Beautiful

The real truth about potentially harmful cosmetic ingredients that are widespread throughout the industry.

ISBN 1-932458-04-2
(4 1/2 x 7)

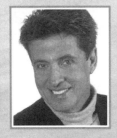

PETER LAMAS

One of the leading makeup artist and beauty experts in the world, Peter's clients read like a Who's Who of Hollywood. Peter is Founder and Chairman of BeautyWalk.com, which is dedicated to helping women realize their potential to be beautiful both inside and out. He regularly appears on television and in the media.

BRONZE BOW PUBLISHING

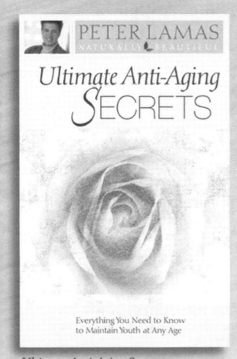

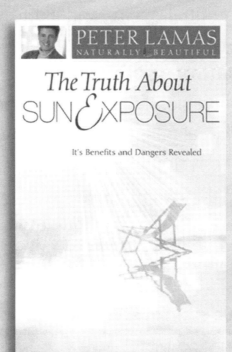

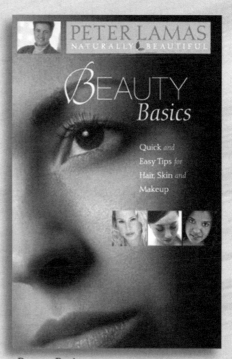

Ultimate Anti-Aging Secrets

Everything you need to know about maintaining youth at any age.

ISBN 1-932458-05-0
(4 1/2 x 7)

The Truth About Sun Exposure

This book reveals the benefits and the dangers of exposure to the sun.

ISBN 1-932458-06-9
(4 1/2 x 7)

Beauty Basics

Quick and easy tips for hair, skin, and makeup.

ISBN 1-932458-07-7
(4 1/2 x 7)

Unleash Your Greatness

AT BRONZE BOW PUBLISHING WE ARE COMMITTED

to helping you achieve your ultimate potential

in functional athletic strength, fitness, natural

muscular development, and all-around superb

health and youthfulness.

Our books, videos, newsletters, Web sites, and training seminars will bring you the very latest in scientifically validated information that has been carefully extracted and compiled from leading scientific, medical, health, nutritional, and fitness journals worldwide.

Our goal is to empower you! To arm you with the best possible knowledge in all facets of strength and personal development so that you can make the right choices that are appropriate for *you*.

Now, as always, **the difference between greatness and mediocrity** begins with a choice. It is said that knowledge is power. But that statement is a half truth. Knowledge is power only when it has been tested, proven, and applied to your life. At that point knowledge becomes wisdom, and in wisdom there truly is *power.* The power to help you choose wisely.

So join us as we bring you the finest in health-building information and natural strength-training strategies to help you reach your ultimate potential.

FOR INFORMATION ON ALL OUR EXCITING NEW SPORTS AND FITNESS PRODUCTS, CONTACT:

BRONZE BOW PUBLISHING
2600 East 26th Street
Minneapolis, MN 55406

WEB SITES
www.bronzebowpublishing.com
www.masterlevelfitness.com

612.724.8200   Toll Free **866.724.8200**   FAX **612.724.8995**